Life Coaching

A Guide to Self-Discovery and Personal Development, Start Living an Awesome Life with No Regret

BY

GARY DAN CLIFFORD

The trademarks that are used are without any consent, and the publication of the trademark is without permission or backing by the trademark owner. All trademarks and brands within this book are for clarifying purposes only and are the owned by the owners themselves, not affiliated with this document.

Contents

INTRODUCTION

Traditional life coaching is a method that allows somebody to identify areas of their lives that need to be changed and then to apply techniques expertly to produce better outcomes in those areas that are missing. Whereas success coaching is a broader focal point of life coaching, where the success coach encourages the individual to define, establish, and achieve personal objectives correctly.

Performance coaching focuses more on tangible and quantifiable goals, for example, corporate, social, academic, and career-relevant objectives. For example, it is easy to determine if your goal is to make a million dollars in a single year, as the goal is measurable if you have met the goal. In other words, the results are measured; you either succeeded or you did not. However, although you're not quite up to your standards, you can still see whether you're on the right track because you can certainly see whether or not you've improved significantly already.

Sometimes success coaching doesn't just involve success but can also help you learn how to adapt to all the overwhelming achievements you already have. We all have learned the tales about famous people who are legendary and then depart from the ultimate profound end as they did not know how to manage their unexpected successes or how to deal with them. A great success mentor will help guide you toward progress. We can help you learn how to push the accelerator quicker and how to accelerate to focus on stability, equilibrium, and resilience.

While it is more general and emotional with life coaching, sometimes the assessment of the tests is not so cut and dry, and a certain level of subjectivity should be measured.

For example, a person may sometimes feel incomplete, and from a particular area of his life, he seeks a feeling of happiness or satisfaction. But how do you define good fortune? It is merely a subjective reaction, which for most people, is unique.

Moreover, great life coaches understand that their clients are the authority in their own lives. Even so, that may not be enough, because sometimes the consumer might be too close to where the best ways to attain dominance cannot be optimized. But a highly trained life coach can more objectively see the situation as a foreign observer, he can utilize his extraordinary abilities to guide the person towards the inside and help them to define the results that make the most sense for the individual and his or her unique situation. Eventually, but not least, a good life coach also brings the best out of your consumer and shows them the right steps to achieve the desired outcome.

Many people have somehow encountered help from an individual that brought out the best of it. Such people influenced your perception and inspired you to step into your dreams. These people often appeared by chance, and they might not even know how much their impact has been in your life, because you probably never told them that. So, what if you could call an extraordinary person like this on-demand to encourage you to take the right steps to help you achieve your fullest potential.

We can be the guiding light for you when you meet Regan Hillier International. We are certified to unleash your grandeur and artfully build and enhance your innate abilities to aid you on your journey to transformation into the absolute supremacy you seek.

In a collaborative effort, we will work together to develop a plan for you so that you will achieve greater security, loyalty, and purpose. Everyone has their definition of success, but our ongoing dedication to professional development and growth will enable us to achieve full potential. Our program gives you the tools to handle some painful periods in your life. Whether you're currently at the top of the mountain, or even feeling stuck or overwhelmed, we will help you achieve the outcomes you want to see in your life. You will finally return by working with us to feel empowered, confident, and happy. It is effortless; anyone who desires achievement; however, you identify this, can get there far quicker with the right coach. It is clear.

CHAPTER 1: COACHING LEADING TO SUCCESSFUL LIFESTYLE

Coaching is the technique of creating an environment, through conversation that facilitates the process by which an individual can move in a fulfilling manner towards desired goals" Coaching becomes a tool for helping people achieve a higher degree of both physical and mental well-being when those aspirations have to do with safety, nutrition, and well-being.

Coaches utilize evocative, more than academic strategies for clients, to build such an atmosphere. We do more to listen than to chat, more to inquire then to say, and more to think than to speak. Coaching does not advise clients on how to solve problems, or inform clients on what to do, or examine the root causes of client dilemma. Although counseling, teaching, or evaluating issues are sometimes a part of coaching, they are neither the primary purpose nor the coaching method. Coaches become constructive and co-creative participants in the efforts of learners to achieve their goals and priorities.

1.1 Why We All Need Coaching?

We all recognize the need for traveling mentors if we want to be safe and well. While most of us are hoping for greater physical and mental well-being, there is considerable evidence that we are moving in the opposite direction and taking the illusion. Despite ongoing media attention to healthy lifestyles, there are now more individuals overweight than the undernourished globally (WHO Fact Sheet, 2006).

The condition in the United States is especially dire. A recent study shows that Americans at the same age and social status are significantly less balanced and more overweight than Brits.

Why are we making the paradox? While obesity is a multifactorial epidemic, at least four factors lead us to choose unwisely quick fixes that don't last, and this endangers our confidence— what psychologists call self-efficacy. Second, there are the daily expectations that have never been rising. Second, we are presented with a bewildering array of recommendations, products, and services on health, making it challenging to build a specific recipe. Second, the difficulty of overcoming the unavoidable obstacles to transition, including uncertainty, reluctance, and ambivalence, is current. Third, a number of us have a recurring history of failure. Most of us don't realize we should control our weight and wellbeing.

We just want to be safe. They love being in control of our well-being and feeling better. We want more strength.

But there is a massive gap between wishing to be well and the daily reality of living with the consequences of overeating, under-exercising, and getting too little space to refresh our battery on physical and mental health.

The evidence is conclusive. Getting slim, reliable, and having a healthy level of body fat are safe and effective revolutionary medicines that help prevent and cure virtually any studied affliction, including mental health.

A quotation from Tal David Ben-Shear, Professor of Positive Psychology at Harvard University, is noteworthy: "not exercising is stressful." Well, dealing with depression and through life satisfaction (e.g., sense of mission, happiness, and meaning) are embracing exercise and eating well as "lifestyle drugs." Two-thirds of health care costs are influenced by our everyday decisions. Yet intelligence doesn't suffice.

Just one in twenty adults were interested in all the top-six well-being habits (Kerrigan, 2003): regular exercise, balanced fat consumption, at least five portions of fruits and vegetables a day, minimal alcohol, non-smoking, and a healthy weight.

Getting people to full fitness is at the core of the physical and mental health practitioners ' hopes and dreams of today. First time in human history it happened that being in charge of one's well-being and making day in and day out wellness decisions are primed to be prevailing social topics, just as smoking cessation or sacrificing for the greater good during World Wars I and II.

Need to Learn A New Life Skill: to build a specific roadmap for well-being and to become assured that we can execute it. Most of us don't believe we will practice this ability in life; the increasing number of those who prefer bariatric surgery is the expression of our most significant reservations.

The health and fitness industry has worked very hard to support us. There have never been more professionals, appraisals, services, guidance, technologies, media, web tools, and beautiful high-tech facilities before.

Though all of these tools are valuable, we need more. We usually ask professionals to advise us what to do, and when we have low self-efficacy, this strategy is not optimal. Doctors are qualified to provide medications and guidance and often strive harder to help us than we do. But in fact, the expert approach lets us off the hook, sending the subtle message: You are not in charge.

The specialist solution is crucial when dealing with an immediate health problem or when we discuss surgery. This comes with a price to assign to experts: we are not in charge, and we are not asked to work and discover our responses.

Building trust needs different patterns of thinking, doing, and relating.

They also need a change of focus to our talents and potential, drawing on what succeeds in our lives and away from the fixation on diagnosing and repairing what doesn't. The more we dwell on the latter, the more that we lose trust in ourselves. It makes change harder, not easier when we focus on what's wrong and what doesn't work. This harvests not enough constructive energy and emotion to drive the process of progress.

Throughout fact, we will have a holistic view of health and well-being. Specialists who specialize in just one field, such as fitness, diet, or mental health, without understanding or connection to the others, are doomed to have little effectiveness or even damage.

Both fields are intrinsically intertwined, and they are dealt with together more effectively. Many people need help combining information from multiple sources to decide what actions to take and how to approach it. It is confusing to people when the specialists dispute each other. This is not a formula to encourage Attitude. "I can do it!"

Another one is there's never significant and lasting improvement without a sincere higher purpose— we need to relate longevity, well-being, and exercise to what we admire most. Third, we need to build a lifestyle program for survival, prosperity, and nutrition that is uniquely adapted to our conditions and capacities.

For a long time, skilled trainers have been known since their ability to support players, sports teams, and managers succeed at their peak. Professional coaches also help clients create meaningful changes in their wellness and well-being.

The new careers in nutrition, health, and fitness are designed to enable people to work efficiently, to overcome obstacles, to improve security and safety, and to make last-minute changes.

With a focus on building auto performance, qualified coaches can be trained to:

• agree and meet where we are today;

• invite us to take responsibility;

• lead us in thinking, feeling and doing work to build trust;

• help to identify a higher purpose for health and well-being;

• reveal our natural impulse to be right;

Help us to tap into our inherent fighting spirit.

1.2 What is a Life Coach?

The life teacher is like a coach. Through supporting other people and showing them aspects of their life where they might need to change or look things differently, they mentor and help people.

Just as a baseball coach teaches you to throw the ball or swing the bat in the right way, a life coach can make you do more of the things that are important to you and do them differently.

Being a life coach is a means of improving others' lives and supporting yourself along the way.

What is Life Coach Doing?

A life coach can do several things in a lot of areas.

As a life coach, you will direct others by attaining targets they never thought possible.

Will help people uncover their guiding values and heal the wounds that hold them back.

Interaction, positive reinforcement, and transparency are critical areas in which a life coach will be involved daily.

Life coaching helps people improve their lives, both personal and professional. Whether they want to enhance their partnership with others, drive their company forward, or have more balance with their life, a mentor will assist in creating, learning, and achieving those goals.

Coaching life keeps individuals responsible and provides them with the resources to see results and change their lives.

1.3 Types of Life Coaches

Just as there are different types of sports coaches, different types of life coaches occur.

What's good with you? What do you want to see people excel?

Answering these questions will help you determine what kind of life coach you're searching for.

1. Career-Life Coach

Usually, a career-life coach is someone who is or has been in a particular industry where coaching is required.

Not only will the career life coaches speak the language of that particular industry, but they will also recognize the kind of mindset needed for that sector. Because they understand what's required, in those spots, they can spot the areas where you are having trouble and make breakthroughs.

Think carefully about the importance you would bring to the table if you want to function as a life coach. Which kind of business did you work in? How long have you been living over there?

You want to give your customers the best possible value, and you can only do that if you can genuinely offer the experience and information that those customers need to succeed.

Almost anyone in any field will profit from a career-life coach.

2. Personal Life Coach

Many people are looking for their own life coach as they believe, like having lifetime support; in fact, it will also benefit them throughout their professions.

They're right, so what's there to offer a personal life coach?

In brief, this sort of mentor is someone who can help someone achieve goals, resolve challenges and difficulties, and make someone find blind spots in life where something important is missed.

They are going to help people when they like. They either can't get ahead or when they hurt themselves. Personal life coaches support people who feel trapped with their lives or are having trouble triggering the Law of Attraction.

It can be gratifying to help people move beyond things that have held them back. Helping someone who might be struggling and assisting people in realizing something about them can also help you understand things about yourself is a satisfaction.

Therefore, you're just making yourself thrive by supporting others.

3. Spiritual Life Coach

A coach of the spiritual life allows you to relate to a higher power.

A spiritual life coach will help you to understand how to better connect with the World so that you can have the most of all that it has to offer. If someone has meditation problems, a spiritual life coach also helps in that area.

4.Business Life Coach

A business life coach is not quite the same. As a company mentor, you're going to show others how to pull in more money and develop the ability to make the right decisions.

Some of the stuff a coach does for a business?

We will build responsibility for their managers. They will come up with actionable proposals. We will help people excel in situations where you may have been lacking in the past.

You can also explain how to network in their profession with others, how to form a group of masterminds, and feel confident as you take your next move.

It's a great way to do more, so work smarter and not harder.

1.4 What Coaching Can Contribute Towards Successful Life?

Becoming a Life Coach doesn't need to be overwhelming. Being a mentor, it will improve life for endless numbers of people.

First of all, you need to be transparent on why we are here and what we should do to support people in accomplishment.

Decide what to achieve. Decide what to sell, and why have the unique credentials to deliver it.

If you are unaware of the answers to those questions, it will be essential to find your reason before starting coaching yourself.

Let's go through what it means to become a mentor and change life...

Inspire people to take action

Coaches present their ideas and concepts in such a way that people will take effect. Ben Franklin quoted, "Tell me, and I forget, teach me, and I may remember, get me involved and learn."

Recognize Emotional Blocks

Coaches help their team recognize their emotional blocks and move quickly through them to get real and lasting performance.

Making A-HA Moments

Professionals simply present knowledge and demonstrate it. But great life coaches are giving those "a-ha" experiences to people.

They speak to all Dimensions of Being a right Person expert talk to a person's head, which means their intellect, their brain. They're offering them the info, directions to do stuff, etc. But a great coach uses a systematic approach of preparation to talk to all seven aspects of an individual's being.

Making Groundbreaking Experiences

Need to build groundbreaking interactions because most of the professionals are overlooked out there. If people go to a seminar, after three or four days, they tend to forget 80 percent of it, and that's if they submit it directly. If they don't apply, then it is more likely they forget almost everything.

Give People an Established System

Consultants and coaches out there just give people information and advice, but transition trainers give people a proven system they should adopt and produce guaranteed results.

Chapter 2: YOUR SYSTEMS FOR LIVING

According to prevailing wisdom, the best way to accomplish what we want in life — getting into better shape, building a successful career, enjoying more and thinking less, is to set specific, actionable objectives.

This is how it usually treats our habits for many years. Each is a task to attain. We set goals for the scores that we needed to go to school, the weights that we wanted to lift in the track, and the income that we tried to make in the company. We've invested in a handful, but a number of them crashed. Eventually, we started to realize that our outcomes had very little to do with the targets we set and almost everything to do with the structures we adopted.

If you are a coach, maybe your goal is to win a championship. The system is the way athletes are hired, the assistant coaches are handled, and you train.

If you're an entrepreneur, maybe your goal is to build a million-dollar business. The program is like checking product ideas, hiring staff, and managing marketing campaigns.

If you're a guitarist, that your goal is to play a new piece, the program is how often you train, how you break down and deal with steep steps, and how the instructor's guidance approach is used.

Now to the interesting question: would you still excel if you neglected your objectives entirely and concentrated only on the system? Of starters, if you were a basketball coach and you overlooked your goal of winning a championship, how would you get results?

The goal in sports is to finish with the best score instead of looking scoreboard and wasting time.

Only getting better every day is the best way actually to succeed. In terms of Bill Walsh, the three-time Super Bowl winner, "The game takes care of itself." The same happens in other areas of life. If you want better outcomes, so forget to set targets. Then reflect on the program.

What does that mean? Were milestones useless? Not. Goals are useful for establishing a course but better for progressing programs. If you spend too much time worrying about your objectives, and not enough time developing your processes, a handful of problems arise.

Winners and losers have the same goals.

Goal setting results from a severe case of the prejudice of success. They focus on the people who end up winning–the winners–and mistakenly assume that ambitious goals contributed to their achievement, thus ignoring all the others who had the same aim but lost.

Each Olympian is trying to win a gold medal. Each worker is trying to get the position. And if successful and unsuccessful individuals share the same goals, then the goal cannot be what distinguishes the winners from the losers. The British Cyclists were not pushed to the top of the sport by the goal of winning the Tour de France. They'd certainly wanted to win the ride before each year— just like every other professional team. The goal was always there. It was only when a system of continuous minor improvements was implemented that they achieved a different result.

Attaining a target is only a quick change.

Consider getting a messy room then set the aim of cleaning it up. If you are gathering the strength to clean up, you'll have a clean room — for now. But if you maintain the same dirty, pack-rat patterns that in the first-place lead to a messy room, you'll soon be looking at a new pile of clutter and waiting for another burst of inspiration.

You're forced to pursue the same goal because you've never changed the system. By addressing the cause, you sent a symptom.

Attaining a target for the moment just changes your life. That's the reverse of change. We believe our findings need to be improved, but the results are not the problem. The processes that produce these outcomes are what we need to alter. If you tackle outcome-level questions, you just briefly fix them. You need to solve problems at the level of the systems to improve for good. Adjust the inputs and adjust the outputs.

Goals restrict your happiness.

The thought behind any goal is this: "Once I reach my goal, then I'll be happy." The problem with a goal-first mentality is that you're continuously putting off happiness until the next milestone. We slid so many times into that hole that we lost count. For years joy has always been something to be enjoyed by my future self. Objectives build an "either-or" conflict: either you achieve your goal, or you struggle, and you're a failure. You lock yourself psychologically into a small definition of joy. That would be mistaken. Your current future course is unlikely to match the precise direction you had in mind before you started. Limiting your happiness to one situation when there are many pathways to achievement don't make sense.

The cure offers a system-first mindset. You don't have to hesitate to encourage yourself to be satisfied when you fall in love with the method rather than the result. Every time your system runs, you can be happy.

And a program in many different forms can be useful, not just the one you first imagine.

Goals are at odds with long-term progress.

Finally, a goal-oriented mindset may create a "yo-yo" effect. Most cyclists work hard for months, so they stop training as soon as they cross the finish line. There's no competition to inspire them anymore. If you spend all of your hard work on a particular goal, what's left to move you further after you've accomplished it? That is why, despite achieving a goal, often people find themselves reverting to their old habits.

Setting targets is about winning the game. Building devices are intended to continue playing the game. Right, long-term thought is a plan without objectives. This is not about any single achievement. This is about the process of continuous improvement and constant refining. It's your interaction with the mechanism that decides your success.

Fall in Love with Systems

Neither of these is to suggest objectives are pointless. It is noticed, though, that targets are perfect for preparing the development, and the processes are useful for making real progress. Plans can guide in the short term and even move you along, but ultimately a well-designed system will always prevail. All matters have a program. It's the contribution to the process that makes the difference.

2.1 The Relationship with the Self

The most important relationship in life is arguably your relationship with yourself. Self-relation is the cornerstone of all else— even altruism. It's easy to identify narcissistic facets of self-relatedness— negative narcissism, excessive guilt for oneself, excessively solipsistic outlooks, an inability to relate and empathize with others, etc.

It is also easy to identify characteristics that we equate with others that are in the right place, behave together, show excellent interpersonal skills, and look effective by traditional meanings, and so on.

It's easy to take things for granted— even being able to focus on you in such a way in the first place is a sign of being very lucky.

For proper development, one's relationship with oneself is crucial. It's about a healthy love of oneself. We know so much about how to respond to themselves from key figures–friends, relatives, teachers, colleagues, and other adults. What's right, and what's wrong— what they like, and clearly what they don't like. Relationships with others form relationships with oneself early in development. Interaction with oneself also has inherent tendencies. As we grow up, how others treat us and how others deal with themselves serve as important factors influencing how we approach ourselves as adults.

We claim that if we have parents who find a good enough compromise for their children's expectations as to how we fulfill their own needs, then hopefully, the children will have a higher chance to grow up to an equally healthy balance. Neither will they overly sacrifice their aspirations and energy for the upbringing of children, nor will they fall into the trap of being negligent in pursuing their activities. Furthermore, how parents balance these self-serving needs in coordination with each other is a crucial model for children who see if they share responsibilities well, given their tenderness— or if there is a negative conflict of feelings about one person not being around enough.

"Self-care is not self-indulgence; it is self-preservation. "Audrey Lorded

Self-care is about self-care and mental health. The friendship that you have with yourself is essential for your well-being and also for establishing healthy and happy relationships with others.

To different people, self-care can look like different stuff. For some, self-care might require time to rest every week; for others, it may sweat it out at the gym, or go out for a ride.

Self-care could go for a walk in one's neighborhood, spend time in nature, or regularly see or talk to friends. Here are a few practices that you can start today that can bring about a meaningful change to improve your relationship:

Invest in yourself.

Spend 15–30 minutes of doing something uplifting you each day.

Try finding reality and exception to what's being said as the inner critic or an outer critic discovers flaws.

Going past self-care

Though, despite all the talk of self-care and self-compassion, mindfulness meditation, self-help, and similar common topics, it's been challenging to pin down what it implies, and what it requires, to develop and maintain a good relationship with oneself. Having a perfect relationship with myself means that while we know we need others in many ways, my relationship with myself has become crucial to making the most of my remaining years through adulthood. We want to step towards a secure attachment to ourselves.

What good relationship can you have with yourself?

This is a list of what has just been observed and come up with. A ton of it is going to be old, which bears a lot of it repeated. Repetitive activities can be easy to drop, even when they are excellent for us because it feels humdrum. Perhaps some of that is a valuable new insight.

1. Set aim and build awareness.

Set the overarching goal of maintaining a good partnership for oneself over the years, with the expectation that what this means may evolve over the years.

2. Prepare for the short, medium, and long term.

As part of being proactive about maintaining a great relationship for you, setting priorities across different time frames is essential. Setting realistic goals and establishing benchmarks and measures are established methods of keeping on the right track for each target. Realize that short-term motivation is often focused on gratification (e.g., feeling fantastic, you started a new class you've often wanted to take), but over time, encouragement becomes less motivating, and more about sustaining behaviors and resisting losing new patterns. Blending experimentation with long term gratification is, therefore, an excellent general formula. The long-term benefits are an opportunity that arrives down the road — often just when you need them — but relying too much on immediate gratification can be simple.

3. Adopt an attitude of curiosity and acceptance.

Recognize the inevitability of change, and generally pleasant to embrace without excessive fear. Only in time do we come to see areas that are truly stable and can define who we and others are to ourselves. Be vigilant, though, of making changes that have not been fully explored, or making decisions that somehow don't look or feel right, or getting stuck in indecision.

4. Prioritize basic self-care.

Rest, sleep, exercise, recovery, leisure, and behavioral behaviors are the pillars of a reliable self-care program. It is essential to be linked to one's body and to provide the body as a good custodian as well as holistically. On top of that, proper care for one's physical needs helps everything else work better and tells us on an ongoing basis that we are concerned with ourselves.

5. Be patient with yourself.

This doesn't imply "letting yourself out of the loop" or shirking responsibility, but it does intend to strive for self-assessment without destructively hostile critique or blame. Individuals are often blameless for self-assessment and self-correction, and more often than not, needless shaming contributes to less effective change. Support blame to the degree that it is inevitable— but strive on being kind and benevolent while being honest and taking responsibility.

6. Try others who suit the goals.

 Besides being with people who treat you kindly, it's nice to have partnerships with others who also try to have a good relationship for themselves, both because they are good models and because you can encourage one another in your efforts. For most of us, it's impossible to avoid toxic people altogether, so manage those relationships carefully.

7. Cultivate positive behavior realistically.

Perfectionism is the victim of positive progress and all-or-nothing thought. Most people that I know want to get it sorted in a short time. This almost always leads to failure and continues a destructive cycle of self-blame, and more "cracking the whip." Much of the time, it falls into the dark place of self-abuse and retribution, which is not a formula for improvement, but sometimes people say it is better than nothing. Though recognizing one's needs for maladaptive defenses and the use of survival they have had is excellent, it is a bad idea to stick too tightly to them. Nonetheless, a degree of dissatisfaction with oneself, being "sick of" how things are or becoming "tired" the same way, always precedes improvement. Setting and delivering on expectations that we can meet is a common and effective alternative.

8. Have a personal crisis plan.

Sometimes we get an evil hand from existence, or we make a decision that we regret and despise.

Having a personal recovery strategy at these moments is important because these are periods in which we are also most likely to slip back on old patterns to excuse self-abuse. The best approach is to anticipate certain moments to arrive and be armed for ways to understand how we feel, which allows us centered on long-term goals and expectations when solving the immediate issue. It can be beneficial to write down our feelings for this eventuality and return to them, and to have a few close people around for those moments to help keep things in perspective. When you realize that at these moments, you prefer to refuse help, stay on top of that because it is the thread that leads everything else to crumble.

9. Maintain constructive activity.

Instead of creating a predetermined definition of success, strive for regular activities that offer pleasure and a sense of achievement. It's necessary to find ways to make it meaningful— this may be about improving what you're doing or working on.

2.2 Awareness: The Gateway Drug to Awesomeness

The subject of self-awareness has been studied by philosophers and psychologists for the last century, from the ancient Greek aphorism "know you" to western psychology.

After all, high self-awareness levels benefit both to oneself, and one's social relations.

What is Self-Consciousness?

Simply put, self-awareness is self-awareness the self-being, which makes one's identity special. These unique components include ideas, experiences, and skills.

The study of self-awareness in neuroscience can be traced back to 1972. The auto-consciousness hypothesis was founded by psychologists Shelley Duval and Robert Wick Lund.

They proposed: "As we reflect on ourselves, we measure and equate our current behavior with our expectations and principles. As objective evaluators of ourselves, we become self-conscious. "Essentially, they consider self-consciousness a significant mechanism of self-control.

It is essential to recognize that self-awareness is not just about what we notice about ourselves, but also about how we see our inner world and monitor it.

Hint: if you ever said, "I should have done it" to yourself, then you know what I mean. Next time you judge something you've said or done, consider the question: "Is what I experienced an opportunity to learn and grow, too? Have other individuals made a similar mistake and learned from it? "Self-awareness goes beyond accumulating knowledge of ourselves: it is also about paying attention to our inner state, with the mind of a beginner and an open heart.

Our mind is exceptionally skilled at storing information about how we react to a particular event to create a template for our emotional life (source).

Such information often ends up our mind to react in some way as in the future, we encounter a similar event.

Self-awareness helps us to be mindful of this mental conditioning and preconceptions, which can form the basis of freeing the mind from it.

Does Self-Consciousness Matter?

It is the ability to monitor our emotions and thoughts from moment to moment, is essential to understand ourselves better, being at ease with who we are, and controlling our thoughts, feelings, and actions proactively.

Furthermore, self-aware people tend to act actively (instead of responding to passively); they appear to be in good psychological health, having a positive outlook on life.

Sutton's investigation (2016) also looked at the parts of self-awareness and its benefits.

The study found that self-reflection, perspective, and perception facets of self-consciousness may contribute to benefits such as becoming a more compassionate individual. In contrast, aspects of rumination and cognition can lead to emotional burdens. Several researches have shown self-consciousness as a crucial feature of successful business leaders.

Self-awareness — was the strongest predictor of overall success in this study.

Self-consciousness is crucial for psychotherapists, too.

"Therapists need to be mindful of their perceptions, ideas, traditional attitudes, and prejudices to represent culturally diverse clients properly" (Oden et al., 2009).

It was also called a "precursor to multicultural skills" (Buckley & Fold, 2010). Self-awareness, in other terms, helps clinicians to understand the differences in their perceptions and the lives experienced by their clients.

This can help psychologists make their clients more non-judgmental and help them understand their clients more.

Why is it hard to be Self-Conscious?

If self-awareness is so essential, then why are we not more self-aware?

The most obvious answer is that we're actually "not there" for studying ourselves most of the time. We are not there, in other words, to pay attention to what is going on inside or around us.

Besides the constant movement of the mind, the different cognitive bias also affects our ability to have a precise understanding of ourselves; we tend to believe narratives that support our already existing sense of self.

Also, confirmation bias may trick us into searching for or interpreting information in a manner that confirms our preconception of something.

Have you had that sensation when you approved a job offer but are still looking for extra proof that this is the perfect job for you? That, in its most beautiful, is confirmation bias.

The lack of willingness to receive guidance might also operate against us if we want a more holistic view of ourselves through others ' eyes.

If we want to develop our self-awareness, how do we balance that with these social patterns in which only those representations of ourselves are recognized?

It's not easy, but some options do exist.

What further complicate the image are the various aspects of the self to which we relate in everyday life.

Daniel Hahnemann, for his contribution to behavioral science, is Nobel Prize winner.

Hahnemann explains in his TED talk the difference between the "experiencing self" and the "remembering self" and how that affects our decision-making.

He states how we feel at the moment about the encounter and how we recall the memory can be very specific and have a connection of only 50 percent.

This disparity can have a significant impact on the narrative we tell ourselves, the way we respond to ourselves and others, and the choice we make, even though most of the time, we might not notice the difference.

Self-Awareness vs. Self-Focused Attention

 For our purposes, let us assume that self-awareness is to be conscious of our personalities and perceptions and how they contribute to those of others.

Self-centered ness consists of just worrying about oneself.

Self-focused behavior, for example, may imply that a psychologist worries about how nervous they are about the therapy session, which causes the person to believe the counselor is not paying attention to them.

In other terms, as one study suggests, "self-awareness could be a method for the negative impact of impeding self-focused attention on self-efficacy therapy." This study provides an essential look at how counselors can change that habit and move towards self-awareness while meeting clients.

It is crucial to be self-aware of all aspects of one's thoughts, rather than be aware of the current emotion one feels.

Some of the techniques that clinicians can use to avoid upsetting self-awareness include continuing to concentrate on the person, their desires, and the therapy session's objectives.

Another approach is to use self-awareness as a means of understanding the customer more, rather than just being self-aware of one's emotions and being overwhelmed.

Anyone who puts time to it can sense the tremendous benefits of high self-awareness.

Techniques of Cultivating Self-Consciousness

Build some space for yourself.

When you're in a dark room without windows, it's pretty hard to see things. The space you create is that crack on the wall where you allow light to pass through.

Stay away from internet media and spend some time by yourself, reading, writing, meditating, and communicating with yourself–maybe first thing in the morning or half an hour before sleep.

Practice mindfulness.

Self-awareness is the secret. Jon Kabat-Zinn describes awareness as "to pay attention in a particular way, consciously, in the present moment, without judgment." In cultivating awareness, you will be more comfortable in yourself, so that you can "be there" and understand what is going on inside and around you. It is not about lying with your legs crossed or hiding your feelings. It's about keeping an eye on your inner state as it arises. You should exercise mindfulness whenever you want by listening carefully, dining conscientiously, or walking.

Keep a newspaper:

Writing not only helps us to process our thoughts but also makes us feel connected to ourselves and at peace. Reading will generate more headspace as well as making your ideas spill out to paper. Research shows that writing down stuff we're happy for or even issues we're dealing with helps improve happiness and contentment. Try this at home–choose a half-day on a Sunday, pay close attention to your inner world–what you hear, what you say yourself, and take note of what you do every hour. You might be surprised to listen to what you write!

Practice well, listening.

'Listening isn't the same as listening. Hearing is about being aware and paying attention to the feelings, body movement, and vocabulary of other people. You'll also be better at listening to your inner voice when you become a good listener by growing your own best friend.

Gain different points of view:

Request feedback. Often, we may be too scared to ask what others think of us— yes, sometimes the comments may be distorted or even deceptive. Still, as you understand more about yourself and others, you will be able to differentiate them from real, sincere, and positive feedback.

Work has shown that receiving 360-degree reviews in the workforce is a useful tool for enhancing self-consciousness (Source) of managers. We all have blind spots, so seeing a fuller picture of ourselves helps gain a different perspective.

Self-awareness is a costly and complicated subject, as "arguably the most fundamental issue in psychology, from both a developmental and an evolutionary perspective."

As human beings, if such a destination exists, we may never fully understand ourselves. But perhaps it is the journey of self-exploration, knowledge and becoming that makes life worth living.

Whether you want to be more self-acceptance or more accepting of others, cultivating self-consciousness is an excellent place to start.

2.3 Listening and Connecting

We had never had any more excuses not to listen. When technology progresses and news expands, we keep spreading our focus through multiple screens, topics, and people — often all at once. As a consequence, publicity has become one of the scarcest–and one of the most important–commodities.

In a culture fractured by noise, those who can listen have a unique advantage. We are not just about stimuli but commitment, not just about contact but attachment. Of course, by listening, we're not talking about "hearing" people, or even tracking what they mean.

Listening transcends awareness. Listening means being fully present with what someone else is saying, processing their words without distraction, and seeking to understand them before attempting to understand ourselves. Hearing is the partnership currency, and the portal of confidence, communication, and reciprocal engagement.

The nature of our interactions, our partnerships, and our reputations all rely on how well this one essential task can be performed.

So, here's our useful Listening Guide.

Practice active listening.

"Have you ever heard me? "You are caught off guard by the question. You were aware, of course, you claim. Yet the other person was feeling the need to ask that question.

People can tell if your verbal responses and your body language make you listen. You give a different message when you're making eye contact and smile as they're interacting than if you're staring into space.

The phrases you use and your body language are part of a more considerable skillset called active listening, a mechanism in which the audience listens to the speaker by consciously interpreting, re-stating, and reacting to what they have learned. For communication and relationships, active listening is crucial. You need to be interested in them, to get someone interested in you.

The most obvious way to respond is through active listening. You already know, for instance, that you have to acknowledge the thoughts of somebody to indicate that you listened. Yet one-word responses, like "yes," "cool," "interesting," or "totally," just telegraph that you usually don't respond to. We are not a statement of substance. People catch on fast. Think back to your last interaction like this, and you know the effect on a friendship that these perfunctory terms bring.

It's easy to develop a great conversation powered by active listening, and it's about listening:

1. Write an open question.

2. Listen to the answer.

3. Follow up with a statement (ideally a public declaration —
but not another issue).

If your concerns sound nonsensical, it's okay. Think back on
fundamentals: Who? What? What? When? When? Where to
go? Why? For what? How? How? All of these are great ways
of starting conversations. For instance, if you're talking about
travel, and the conversation has a lull, you might just ask a
random question. That may sound strange or unnatural, but
you'll be surprised at how ordinary it is. Hardly ever long
conversations.

Talk on an emotional level.

 A lot of people (especially men) listen on a logical level. Look,
this is the simplest way to guide a conversation, and it is often
the safest. It is not unnatural, then.

If you want to communicate with someone, however, you'll
need to respond to them on an emotional level.

This is crucial to the development of meaningful relations.
You show empathy when you respond to someone in an
emotional way. They know as they empathize that someone
else is just as important as you are. Understanding is one of
the most endearing and emotionally resonant interactions that
you can have with someone else. Yet from a young age,
several adolescents are deliberately instructed to suppress or
conceal their feelings, or unwittingly tend to do so.

. Men pay less attention to their opinions, and so therefore
often pay less attention to the emotions of others. They find
empathy hard to find. We have no scope or closeness to their
marriages because they have no emotional connections.

That's fine. It needn't be like this. Here's how you stay back in
touch with your feelings and empathize with the other people:
there's a feeling attached to it behind all that someone asks
you, whether its reality or beliefs

. Logical relations are about finding common ground and shared interests. Neither are personal bonds. And that is great because emotions are the one last thing that connects us all. Each of us may have passed through different things, but we all shared the same feelings.

Share moments in your life where you have felt the same emotions to build up an emotional connection.

They're going to be uncomfortable. If you don't speak much about your history, current, or future, you'll probably realize that people in your life aren't willing to share it. Building relationships and emotional connections are challenging without being a bit vulnerable first and sharing your narrative first. Show your emotions, provoke your emotions, and then connect the two.

I'll tell the story of my father passing away and my girlfriend breaking up with him when I teach in our Residential Boot camp. The worst part: Both of these things occurred within eight months. After that, I ask the guys that I'm coaching to choose from this tale one emotion that resonated with them and tell a story of their own based on that emotion. Half of the guys continue, "My friendship with my daughter..." or something similar, "My wife..." See what happened there?

The men went right for the father's rational point of contact. However, it was not an intense one. What about the pain, sorrow, and sadness? Perhaps thankfulness, or remorse, or guilt? You must activate the emotions that come through.

This takes a bit of time to get into your emotions and to connect personally with other people. When you fail at first, don't panic because it will come with time. Best of all, you'll notice that your friendships and relationships are getting more profound and more productive.

Keep on asking the other person.

"What do I mean now? "Perhaps one of you has accidentally touched upon a sore subject or just dried up the conversation. The other party may just go to the bathroom and returned. Or perhaps you sense this person's need to please, as you know that they are becoming increasingly important to you. Either way, lulls in discussions will lead you to fly two steps over your own. Here's how you can stop that: You don't care when you're concerned about the "right" thing to say. If you were, that'd focus your brain on what the other person was saying. So, whenever you start to worry about what to ask next, this is a useful reminder to engage in the discussion.

If you've ever been in a discussion on the receiving end of that, you'll know how annoying–and bright–it's. Just ask yourself questions, instead, if you catch yourself doing that.

For example, you can ask yourself:

What is this person saying?

How does that person feel about what they're thinking about?

How did I mean, is close to what they're talking about?

How did I feel this way?

Asking questions will prevent a common mistake that is focused on yourself rather than others. It sets the stage for you to establish an emotional connection with somebody (more about this in a sec).

Just note, their tale will take precedence over your narrative. Problems prohibit you from thinking about yourself. It may sound simple and straightforward, but when you catch yourself worrying about a lull or making an excellent first impression next time, ask yourself questions so you'll be prompted to listen. Thought about what the other individual was doing, and hear.

Pay attention to how they pronounce it.

You may already have noticed statistics showing that most of our correspondence is performed without words (estimates vary between 60 to 90 percent).

You listen to gestures, their speech, their pronunciation, and look at the vocabulary of their body and how it moves. All of these images will give your insight into their emotions and what they mean. That's why email and instant messages are so confusing, and why when you listen to someone, you need to be fully present.

Create your exposure to shifts in their vocabulary of expression and body. Look at how they articulate themselves:

Will the other person's speech sound higher? Perhaps the subject makes them nervous, or it brings up an unpleasant memory.

Should they speak quicker, or do they stutter more? You might have stumbled at something they're passionate about, and there's so much they can't keep up to say their mouth.

Do they avoid eye contact? You could have broached an uncomfortable subject.

When you appear to imitate the other individual instinctively, then how does your body language make you feel? At first, it won't be easy, but as you pay more attention and get the feedback, you'll be able to pinpoint more precisely how exactly someone feels when they're talking.

You can also make use of quiet moments and pauses to get more clues about how someone feels. If they are interested in continuing a discussion with you, so their natural reaction is to ask a question and get to know. If they aren't, well, the quiet may last longer than you would have been comfortable with.

Sparingly using humor.

A lot of people try to get funny too hard. We push laughter when there is little. Yet humor breaks the emotional tension built up. Though you may consider friction stressful and unpleasant, if you use it correctly, it can be equally powerful. As our podcast guest, Oren Cliff, states, "Stress is what keeps people's attention." By removing the stress, you allow more productive, more difficult emotional discussions.

You could be humorous, for example, when the other person attempts to talk about something that means a lot to them. They're going to feel like you don't take them seriously or are real with them. You didn't mean to say it, but it does make them feel like that. Sometimes on your end, it's a defense mechanism to avoid the emotional connection and to avoid getting hurt.

Resist the impulse to continually joke about in the more severe or tense moments of a conversation. Alternatively, listen to the words and tonality, and recall how they sounded when you did.

Closing Thoughts

Dig into learning comprehension and rational links. Create an emotional connection so you can feel empathy for the other person and get a sense of how they think.

Don't be getting crazy about what you're going to be doing. Then, get your attention back to the moment of issues that play before you. Look out for their body language and the words. Pay attention, and let the times of dangerous, uncomfortable, or awkward interaction pass. Sometimes the most beautiful can be the painful or intense portions of a conversation.

The first or second time you're listening, you might not get it entirely. Keep on. You are going to get the hang of that. And you will know how satisfying that might be.

2.4 Choices and Decisions

While it may seem that the words "choice" and "decision" are merely synonyms of the same thing, there is a difference between the two.

We learn from empirical experiments that the disparity derives from the principles of liberty and determinism, where independence is the place of choice and determinism is the point of judgment.

Determinism is the doctrine that ultimately determines every event in its complete form, including human action, by causes external to the will. So, we can't choose anything. All was decided.

Choice, on the other hand, if it is pure, implies just what you believe it does: the right to choose among various alternatives, without being limited by other requirements and constraints. None of this was decided.

So, are the determinists right, that everything is predetermined? Probably not, although we must admit that decisions are usually influenced by factors external to them. Likewise, absolute freedom is rare — constraint is the norm, in some form or another.

Don't race to a decision point. Reconnect first to the place of choice.

Ethical decision-making can only come from a given location. To get there, you have to make a conscious effort to rid yourself of anxiety and perceived limits. You have to open your mind to all possibilities, without having to feel restricted. Everything seems like an insurmountable problem when you're in there. Instead, there are only opportunities for development and exploration. None of that can stop you.

Crossroads between feeling fulfilled and aligning with your values are the place of choice. You can only step on to the point of judgment after you have established the position of choosing, which is where you consider all options and determine what to do.

Let's use a remote TV, as an illustration, to demonstrate. You have the right to choose from an infinite list of shows and networks with your App. You might go for a basic comedy, a science TED talk, or a golf tournament. You are at the right place to choose.

Yet, you're not making decisions in a vacuum. Your preferences are affected by a multitude of external and internal influences, such as habit, history, employment, ambitions, etc. It is when you start to take these factors into account that you move to the decision point.

So, if you're only watching TV for fun, then a basic comedy or reality show may just be perfect. If you want to be able to take part in the workplace small talk the next day, though, you can choose a curriculum you know your friends will be thinking about.

We don't talk about the process of making this judgment. We just do it instantly. Nonetheless, it is believed that if you slow down and evaluate the cycle, you can achieve better results not only in deciding which TV show to see but also with the critical decisions in your life.

Another example: You're about to hire a new employee and have a variety of eligible applicants. You can choose among any of them at the place of choice. One is exactly as good as the other. Nonetheless, we will take into account the requirements of the company, the qualifications, backgrounds, etc. of each applicant. This is the place of the decision—-where all relevant factors have limited our possible choices.

That is the fundamental distinction between preference and judgment. Choice connects to the desired place of intent, values, and beliefs. Decision connects with the area of behavior, performance, and effect. One may claim preferences are linked to motives, and actions are linked to triggers.

Understanding the difference between the position of preference and decision point lets you practice defining your emotions, whether positive or negative, so you can create motivated choices and make simple, comprehensive decisions. You can get the trust needed to stay inspired and take positive, life-changing steps by visiting the place of preference first.

You can avoid regrets about what you have done or not done in life by understanding the difference between choosing and making decisions. Use your full human capacity and be the best possible version of yourself. Understand and appreciate the distinction between decision making and selection.

CHAPTER 3: RECODING YOURSELF: TRANSFORMING YOUR INNER WORLD

Live a lifetime, knowing nothing is guaranteed. This awareness will help you to live life fully. Whatever happens in your life has a purpose, even though that is a painful experience. Believe that it will evolve great things.

Many citizens in the present world are struggling for inner peace. To holy places, they go in pursuit of healing, books of self-help, spiritual retreats, and still cannot find it. The only area that one sometimes forgets to search in is internal. On the contrary, we appear to do the exact opposite.

In moments of silence, we run away from spending time with ourselves, being alone. At that given moment, we hold our minds busy with items that do not serve any purpose. For example: when driving, reading a newspaper, chatting on the park's cell phone while walking, checking Facebook, What Sapp, and the list goes on. This inability to control and calm one's mind leads to stress, anxiety, worry, fears, insecurity, and lack of peace.

We all want to feel happier and freer, but how many are working for it? Inner peace is not a peaceful environment; a complete change of inner world is the magic within.

The key to finding it is not going against nature, just allowing things to flow naturally the way they are supposed to move instead of struggling and manipulating them. You need to trust and understand that whatever happens in your life, even if it is a painful experience, has a purpose. Believe that, through that, great things will unfold. Most citizens refuse to surrender because they don't want to let go, which adds to inner turmoil.

Look out over everything. See how the sun rises, how a caterpillar turns into a butterfly, how the tree sheds its leaves naturally. We all represent the undoubted recognition and submission that we must imbibe in our lives.

Often people who pass in their sleep are happy and leaving everyone surprised. One would like you to spare a moment and think, what if these people knew uncertain life is? What would their standard of living be? How would they have lived with that sort of consciousness? Would they still indulge in frustration and find fault, self-pity, ego, past, or future living? Would they even waste a fragment of their energy in arguments, struggles, forgiveness, or materialistic wishes?

The answer lies in no. So why it that we take our lives for is granted? Might we live forever? Isn't it amazing to still be living, to have another chance to rectify past mistakes and make a change for the better in the world?

Inner transition ideas

Work at the time. Take it the way it comes every day. Do not let past or future energies prevent you from unwrapping the gifts of the present moment and enjoying them.

Start your day with awareness that life is uncertain and that today I have to do my best. Be vigilant about your actions and thoughts.

Out of self-acceptance comes inner peace. It takes on your imperfections as much as it does your perfections. Focusing on and boosting your assets.

Stop comparing your life to others, and graciously accept your lot. Understand that nobody's life is perfect and, behind any closed door, there's a different story.

Choose to be genuinely grateful and caring rather than finding and managing mistakes with others.

Learn how to detach from the past and from the emotions that weigh you down. Let go of thoughts that do not serve any purpose.

Prevent addictions, such as mobile phones and gizmos, which drive us further away from ourselves.

Don't get so worried about life. Learn to laugh in every situation, and find humor.

Spend time in solitude, and respect your true self.

3.1 Rewrite Models of Reality

Every single one of us has a tale about who we are and why. We often have a couple of. These stories express our belief in what we can do and who we believe we can be. They define who we are.

Stories can be useful. Narratives like "I am brilliant with numbers," "Children love me," or "Art is my calling" will motivate us to cultivate and offer our best gifts; they enable us to show up in our relationships with others positively and authentically.

However, our accounts often have less-salutary effects.

Worse, it's they are. Since they (fakery) say that the way things are is because of whom we are, they leave little room for improvement.

Generally speaking, we don't deliberately compose our stories-of-self. When we are kids, they are typically formed, often as coping mechanisms.

"We are all creating stories to explain the events that have felt traumatic or even difficult in our lives," explains psychiatrist Gail Salts, MD, in her book Becoming Real.

For instance, if a parent dies or leaves home, she says, a child may create a story he needs to be left behind.

Or if a girl is caught stealing a candy bar and identified as a juvenile offender, she may be motivated to accept the troublemaker role as a central element in her identity.

Kids in their story making aren't rational; they're only trying to make sense of difficult situations. But these myths can stay embedded in our unconscious minds and influence our actions as adults directly.

Some values which were necessary, rational, and possibly valid at the moment they were developed will later become tremendous restricting forces. A conviction like "Anger is bad," for example, will help a child lie low and stay safe in a tumultuous household.

These often derive from interactions such as possessing a supremely talented parent, and by contrast, these often sound like a second-fiddle failure.

These encounters, in and of themselves, need not characterize us, says Christopher Hall, Ph.D., an associate professor and specialist in narrative psychology at the University of North Carolina Wilmington.

"Things have no significance implicit in them," he notes. One individual may view the master cooking of her father as evidence that she is not material for the kitchen, while another might feel born to cook because her parent was so talented.

Hall argues that what counts is the sense we offer our history. This is how they build our tales. So, when we choose to reinterpret past events to make our position in the better, things change.

"A breakup or any other kind of traumatic occurrence allows you the ability to describe yourself as a perpetrator or survivor," Hall says. "You have the choice ability. We all have that power. "

See Your Story

Our stories that generate identity are made visible mainly by their effects. Look at the life you created, and the patterns you played out. Note the scenes that seem to be the most meaningful and defining within your autobiography. Write them down or say them loudly, and start listening to such elements as:

Negative Self-Talk

Typically placing oneself down or concentrating on your shortcomings may imply that you have an inner tale of indignity. Only seemingly harmless comments such as "I've never been coordinated" or "I'm just not cut out for [fill in the blank]" that suggests that you've got a story that restricts or disempowers you.

Disproportionate Reactions

When you blow your head because the dishes were not done by your friend, she notes, you may add a bigger meaning to a little frustration. And that's an indication it has ignited any inner narrative.

That story could be "your partner doesn't love you or care about you," she says. And if that tale interacts with a larger narrative about how no one will ever really accept you, or that you don't deserve to be cherished, she mentions that even the tiniest mistake or indication of abuse will act as "evidence" that such stories are real— rendering dirty dishes far more disturbing than they need to be.

Repeatable Patterns

Almost always, our external circumstances represent our stories about what is possible. This is why, even when we change jobs, we might end up playing the same part in all our partnerships or witnessing the same aspects of life.

"If you always have partnerships where you're damaged or rejected," says Christine Hassle, MA, Expectation Hangover's life coach, and founder, "then you might have an inner story like' people leave me.'" If you're always dealing with finances, you might have a story that's lousy money or that you don't merit abundance content. "What occurs outwardly is always a product of what's going internally," she notes. "That's why exploring and updating your beliefs regularly is important."

Questioning Reality

Noticing the situation is the first step but it seems unachievable until you explore the inner workings of your storyline. Journaling can be an incredibly effective way to dig into unconscious thoughts and tell the stories that drive us.

Byron Katie, a teacher of the self-inquiry method The Work, recommends that we write down and systematically challenge our judgments concerning our actual reality as a means to unravel our underlying belief.

"The way to end our frustration is to explore the reasoning behind it," Katie says, "and anyone can do so on their own with a sheet of paper and a pen." Once you've found what's sounding like a core belief in your journaling session, sit down with another piece of paper to answer the following questions about it: Katie then advises "turning the narrative around" — retelling various con. You can find your old story less accurate and non-negotiable than you thought after taking on some alternative realities. You might also learn specific things you might be able to tell, stories that make you safe to enjoy a life of your own.

Change Your Story

The area of story therapy offers a blueprint for exposing and reworking tales that may screw with your subconscious, the personality — and existence.

Here's how it functions.

Take a look back:

One of the first objectives in narrative therapy is to "externalize" individual tales, enabling us to analyze and question them. That's not a fast fix. It takes time and space for reflection, and permission to look differently at the events in your life.

Narrative therapy specialist Christopher Hall calls this "definitional room." At its heart, he explains, it's about understanding that "there are a lot of different ways of seeing stuff," and that you can have a choice in how you want to see them.

In many instances, clinicians such as Hall help clients see a more caring and motivated side of themselves and their decisions.

"There is a very western idea that we get stronger by constant self-criticism," Hall says. But by diminishing or marginalizing our successes and overemphasizing our perceived failures and traumas, we are growing the confidence we have in our inherent capability.

Review the tale incrementally: Simple, gradual acts are more successful than large, drastic affirmations in shifting negative stories.

If you're spinning too far on the pendulum, warn life coach. If circumstances don't magically change, you're likely to go back to your old story.

"Create a reasonable story you can grow into, such as:' I'm committed to getting better with money, and I'm as capable of managing a budget like anyone else.'" This could motivate you to take a class or read a budgeting book, which can give you the practical skills you need.

Seek sustainable sources of motivation:

Frequently, its negative experiences— breakups, bankruptcies, self-treaty— that leads us to investigate our stories first. But it turns out that for lasting change, positive feelings and aspirations have much better fuel.

Feelings of vulnerability, anxiety, and pride were powerful key motivators for improvement.

Change your environment:

Given that our stories are often reinforced or triggered by familiar people, and places, a change of environment can provide an excellent setting for your new account to begin.

Part of the advantage of new environments is that they give you some leeway to try new versions of yourself, just as Fuseli Ford did when she went to school. But you'll also benefit from distancing yourself from a whole lot of ingrained habits and triggers.

Note stress effects on your story: Pressure makes us more vulnerable to negative thinking, and more likely to slip into old patterns. Lombardo recommends you question yourself, on a scale of 1 to 10, how depressed you feel the moment you find an old story rearing its unhelpful head. If you're at or above level 6, put brakes on.

"Stop listening to the story and do something healthy and helpful," she says.

"It might take a few deep breaths, do some pushups, go for a walk, and catch a video that makes you laugh, or embrace somebody. There's something that will dial back distress so you can start redefining your reality.

Stand tall: Research shows that merely shifting the attitude and pose could have a drastic impact on your perspective.

Amy Cuddly, Ph.D., a social psychologist found that by standing in a "power pose"— wide stance, broad shoulders, hands-on-hips

a person's testosterone and cortisol levels can change in just two minutes. Such factors are correlated with emotions of control and stress, respectively, and high-power posers did significantly better in simulated work interviews in her experiments than low-power posers.

Cuddly advises that you follow a strength posture a few minutes before every traumatic event. You might even pursue the technique if an old-story reel begins to play in your head.

Ultimately, the goal is to enjoy your life, free and in the moment, without having to have any story.

3.2 Bend Reality

Well, while being a reality bender is a thing, keep in mind that free-will is also one, meaning you can bend reality in whatever direction you choose.

Although things do not need the permission seal to occur, without it, the fact cannot happen.

To be able to be, it requires your feedback. Some might assume there's only one truth, and for everyone, it must be the same. Otherwise, it's just a dream, an illusion, but is it? Sure, it is based on actual evidence but much more like a script than a documentary.

The way you treat anything that occurs has a profound effect on your life, for the good and the bad. Ask your siblings about their childhood if you are still unconvinced and see if their description matches. Whatever happens around us will always go through our eyes before it reaches our brain, where it is recorded as a fact, so it becomes apparent that our perspective can have a substantial influence on the so-called events. Circumstances alone mean little. To exist as a memory, they must be interpreted by us.

If we don't notice anything, it could never have happened. They just aren't part of our lives and our reality. You had to go through all these hypothetical (very detailed) situations and pretend they were happening to be well informed if they were going to happen. It's like solving a thousand mysteries that will go right into the garbage once you've finished it. How many times did all those dreadful things that you dreamed happen? Is there a point in trying to get an answer to a question that still needs to be asked?

Those mental simulations are proven to be able to trigger the same muscle response, brain activity and hormonal discharges that the actual event would trigger, so I decided not to volunteer to star the scary movies that anxiety insisted on playing before my eyes and wait to see what would actually happen and then decide whether there was any need to pull my hair out. The excessive noise and all the talk always made me a bit uncomfortable, so "space out" was quite common for me. The combination of having too many kids with having one that wasn't very attentive to what the rest of the family were up to culminated quite often with me getting lost.

We all had a lot of fun, there were popsicles and swing sets, there were sunlight and music, and there were macaws in a big cage out in the field. Did you ever see any? They are spectacular creatures. For anyone, let alone a child, those bright blue, purple, yellow, and green feathers can be quite hypnotizing! Those big, talkative, colorful birds fascinated me, and it stood there, looking at them because God knows how long.

When the spell was finally broken, the next thing I remember was to look around me and not be able to locate a single member of my vast family. Take Things As they are, it is always told us to stay in the last place where we saw each other, never move around, or it would be more difficult for them to find unfortunately for me the bench was in front of the monkey's enclosure.

What determines whether our Heads go on inside?

There was a moment when I got lost with my older sister at a store.

We should be about seven and nine, and this turned out to be a different experience.

My sister screamed, she started running around the room, searching the halls frenzied with emotions–she ran away as fast as she could so that I couldn't see she was weeping–blurring her vision.

This didn't take her long until she gave up the role of "big sister" entirely and went from silent cries to shamelessly bawl her eyes while pointing out to me how excited all the other kids were trying to hold hands with their dad.

It is not sure whether it was because it was so much more seasoned in getting lost or if it wasn't about being a worrier, but when she came to the point of thinking how our life would be in an orphanage.

Of course, they did. Once we reached the counter, they declared us, and that was the end of it, but the fact is, she was traumatized to get lost just once in a way.

In carefully selecting the viewpoint, we will create something or ruin it.

It's not hard to comprehend the idea, just swipe through your Integra pictures and then link it to one of those influencer pages.

Even though you both have Frappuccino photos in there, perhaps only one of you was fortunate enough to get that extraordinarily beautiful, incredibly delicious version.

If It had been doubled over it and started to analyze all the reasons that could have led to it and the many other subsequent event that Is found unattended

, It might end up feeling bad but honestly, there is so much more to them and our relationship than they were unable to keep us all in check, at all times when we were children that it was just woo

Many variables make up any given situation, and the ones that we decide to focus on in each case are those that will determine how we feel about it.

And if our choices are to push the scales of how we feel about an event, would it be safe to say, instead of the case itself, that you can choose the fact or at least change it with thoughts alone in your favor?

Looking for beauty in any situation is, in my opinion, the best way to bend reality in our favor, and think beauty is everywhere, even in pain.

You may argue that it's easier to say than done, but the truth is that we think it's because it's too easy, too simple that we can't always do it.

Think about it. If there are both things, why would anyone choose ugliness over beauty, fear overconfidence?

Maybe it's because we like to view ourselves as complex beings, live in a complex world, trying to solve complex problems if we want to keep at least a little balance in the center of the mess, but then again, maybe it's just you, doing what you do best.

3.3 Live In Blissipline

Blissipline is a mixture of Love and Discipline. The term is used as you strive to achieve your goals (which take discipline) in the context of being in the now (bliss).

You are no doubt following your objectives with grim determination with blissipline, or using anxiety to inspire you. Instead, there's cheerful energy behind all you do. You are in the present, and the steps toward your goal are the happy journey, not a means to an end.

It takes real courage to dig deep within yourself and find out your true vocation in the workforce and your personal life, including ambition, intention, values and prerogatives, and then picture it as if it would indeed come true. Your real honesty and borders with your life will be even easier to protect until you realize what it is! Can we break it down?

Passion carries risks. It's something that we think about sincerely and typically born from pain or somehow the experience of misery. Translated, the term passion implies "to suffer." By awakening the most active part of our nature and stirring up the wild mustang in our soul, our love gives raw energy and strength to suffer through to fulfill the purpose of calling our hearts and souls.

Purposeful risk is used to harness our passion's wild horses and give them the right direction (let's hope) and rich meaning. They stand for something beyond contentment with the sensory or ego. Rather than saying, "Does that feel good? What am I going to get, or what am I going to lose?" The right risk-taker is asking," How literally wills this risk change the world?" Principles are threats regulated by a collection of necessary as well as moral principles. Chances are simply just choices, and when confronted with critical judgment, values shape a set of criteria for assessing the risk. The ideals of truth, justice, independence, liberty, mercy, compassion, and responsibility are the principles.

Pure exercise of sovereignty and responsibility for your decisions is a prerogative. The right to choose is, in essence, a luxury hard to think of in a spoiled rotten society embedded in the greed in which we reside.

It is by design that we use our sixth sense of experience to decide what challenges are necessary for us in finally creating a life "as the ultimate dream come true." Did I even lose you?

Imagine that you've had a fortune cookie that revealed the Ultimate Magic Formula for Success & Prosperity given your Passion, Intent, Values, and Prerogatives because it's a fortune cookie I have to say, "In Sleep" for good luck after it! (. But every day, the magic mojo formula starts and ends out of your bed.

With the 4 P in mind, first thing before you get out of bed, then hurry until you close your eyes at night with a race "to-do list" for tomorrow, consider this!

First, write down in detail about 5-7 "dreams come true," if you can. To me, this aspect has been super hard to do. Be patient and keep pace with yourself; the aim is just to continue to practice the steps.

Third, (in bed), just concentrate on steady, deep respiration. To stop the noise in your brain, use a Jedi-mind trick to focus a ticking clock or your pulse. Breathe in slowly through your nose five counts; keep your lungs tightly open as far as you can for five counts, exhale emptying your lungs for five counts. Think that you are the Green mile man who purges all the yucky from your anus. Rinse and repeat at least seven times or until fully relaxed.

Second, just after breathing and as long as your feet hit the ground, hop around like a loony-ton for a full song that encourages you to go! Instead, at your reflection in the mirror, SMILE for five counts how crazy you just felt like a loon J Forth hopping about, emphasis on Gratitude by thankful for every little thing you remember! Example: Thank you for this room, and for staying there.

Thank you for showering with clean water, a toothbrush and toothpaste, a packed toilet, clean clothes, coffee, appreciate the beautiful roses while you walk the dog. praise your car for getting you to work safely, tires for staying active on the highway, gas in the tank, food readily available, music on the radio, paying for work to do, friends talking to, complimenting and acknowledging people you're typically passing by; "That's a great color on you, Janet!" Creating genuine compliments creates serious" MOJOY!

Fifth, focus on making Good Affirmation to yourself and others. Yeah, nip the inner mean voice in the booty, the very second a negative thought tries to enter your lovely brain! Take the mean thinking and turn it into a constructive one right away. This is a simple, noisy game to do too! I find myself telling myself, "no, that's stupid" in passing thoughts. So now, I roar to the inner voice when it's about to happen, "Yes! This is a GENIUS!" Which usually splits me up, which is another good thing to do for brain health anyway - a lot of laughter?

The brain is a large lump of fleshy bumpy lumps and zapping lights with nothing within. It is a recording device that does just what your voice is asking you to do and do, not vice versa. Unfortunately, like an evil pet parrot you inherited, it'll do and feel exactly what you're telling it. All that to say, please carefully use your power of thought! Talk to yourself as if you were the most cherished first love, best friend, gentle, loving, continually being a honeymoon lovey-dovey-get a room with your brain "you are so amazing, I love you so much."

Sixth, gets your imaginative visualization going. At first, this is not easy, and I'm still trying to do it as if the mental image I'm creating has already come true.

If you're addicted to looking into the past to define your future (like I was), this will be like the first-time workout expect lactic acid. You may render this a visually enjoyable storytelling period or a private journaling activity but be as ridiculous about it as you like a beautiful fairy tale story in either.

The key is dreaming big but remaining unattached to the outcome. Focus on the life-like Relationship, Money, Fitness, Job of the big area build the high-level visual image of yourself and then narrow it down to as realistic as you can render it "in a beautiful vision come true" universe and let the imagination soar. Imagine what you wear, who you are with, what the surroundings look like, what you smell, and what you taste? Seek to perceive the emotions actually with all six senses, perception being of necessity the 6th sense. This creates a belief in your mind and a way of knowing that, in turn, reality within your heart that illuminates your brain creates new brain switches, which ultimately creates your reality and world experience. That is the underlying principle of quantum physics concerning neuroscience. Dr. Joe Dispense will learn more about that.

Seventh set clear goals daily for your' ideal' day. Setting the goal that everything is going to go well, or even if you anticipate it all to go wrong = you're going to be right!

Eighth, give condolences and blessings to 5 individuals or more. If you're like me, random people appear in my mind through my day, so just take a moment to give them a blessing or quick prayer that focuses on using only positive words. If they are sick, then pray that they will be healed. If they are seeking a job, hope that today they can obtain excellent opportunities and interviews.

Ninth, so far, it's my favorite because it's the most tangible for me to grasp. Hold a pen handy to keep a serendipity running list all day long.

These can be coincidences, freebee's, big and small wins, aha moments, the perfect song at the perfect time, a networking connection referral, a free webinar email about a subject you're involved in, beautiful things people did for you like to hold the door open while your hands were full, etc. You'll be amazed at how easily remembering the sweet little moments that happen all day long makes you immediately satisfied and gives you energy and a mega boost! Appreciation by providing a sincere joy and eagerness to the things you take for granted continues to expect marvelous things to show up and a reminder to pay for it.

Last but not least, pay close attention to what is starting to happen! Agree that what we are focused on in our thoughts and energies is like feeding the wolf tale. When we concentrate on creating new dreams to begin to come true, we just need to imagine it, live it through our six senses, and begin to pay attention to what starts to appear! You remember how "they say".... "Would have eaten you if it were a snake!" Unquestionably paying attention to the clues that are dropped in my path, putting the pieces together in the puzzle is easily the most fun mind game I've ever played!

3.4 Create a Vision for Your Future

"The touchstones of our protagonists are fantasies," once wrote Thoreau, a man who believed in his creativity. A view is the most significant visual or subconscious representation of you. It can also be a set of long-term goals and dreams. A dream determines the ideal optimal future state; it shows you what you'd like to do over a more extended period. Vision can be an own "why" or the intrinsic intent of the life of the organization.

Vision and mission might often be portrayed together. These aren't the same though we may confuse the two at times. There's a crucial difference, though: opposed to dream, the goal is explaining the status quo, what you're doing right now. It is customized to your current capabilities. Your mission determines your organization's current state and work.

Of illustration, consider Space; their goal is: "Space develops, produces and launches innovative rockets and spacecraft." Where a plan explains the now, a dream forecasts the potential future instead. Space thinks that humanity needs to be a multi-planetary species to survive many more generations to come. Accordingly, their goal is "enabling people to live on other worlds." Therefore, by bringing down the cost of rocket launching while operating every day on their task of creating reusable rockets, they ultimately allow more people to be transported and lived on Mars and beyond –which is their specific view of the future to date.

What a Dream Can Do for You

Describe what you are doing now appears potentially helpful. People just want to know what you're doing. But why are you meant to have a vision? For two purposes, each individual or organization should have a dream:

First, you are motivated by an idea, and you give energy. It leads, and ultimately provides meaning to all your efforts. Coming to terms with your "why" connects and roots you to your core values. Your perspective unlocks your deepest motivations. Making the connection between your core principles of heart and your daily work would render you invincible.

Second, it controls a system of decisions. This helps you to reflect on what to do (and not do) in the potential for those successes five, ten years, or more.

Once the dream and priorities are straightforward, it's easier to say yes wholeheartedly or say no with an acceptable reason.

Finding and Developing Your Very Own Vision

When you're looking for your vision, it's best to do that offsite somewhere you're inspired and not distracted. Think about someplace more relaxing as a little secluded lodge in the mountains or by the sea, rather than your workplace. A central question when it comes to building your dream is, "What is my Why?" If you think of this, what are the hopes that you have just started working on, or that you should finally start working towards? Simon Sine's book Begin with why each individual or company needs to know why to get the rest (what and how) corrects and figured out. Which ensures you'll quickly find out the and how later if you know the Why? Zoom out, and focus on your picture's most giant, long-term version.

Respect the following criteria when formulating your vision:

Unique: make sure it fits in with your passion and values and is unique to you. Which involves seeing yourself in part, too? So, what do you look like in that role three years from now? How do you see one another?

•Write it directly, so that it is quick to grasp and can be easily repeated at any given time by any employee.

Focused: Narrow in so that it is not too broad.

Bold: Are they brave enough and big enough? Stretch out instead of staying inside the quo.

Beneficial: A good vision always has a reason and, at the same time, strives to benefit not only you but others too. For example, a company will support its clients first but, at the same time, still, help you or your affiliate. Profit is the product of outstanding service, not a target in itself.

Aligned: The dream and approach to it should be matched, but most notably, they should not dispute one another for purposes of validity. Of starters, an organization that wants to change the world often fundamentally requires policies and guidelines that are constructive on the inside.

Inspiring: Write the impetus to your dream. Think of a sci-fi film trailer that pulls millions into the cinema; it should have a strong magnetic pull to your goal.

Engaging: Creating an idea is like building a house: you may not know how to make a house yourself, but you have thoughts and pictures in your head that you are passed on to an artist who helps you develop drawings and plans to build and produce the final product. Overall, you hear an excellent vision once and never forget it. It will help you achieve that goal by respecting these criteria.

Applying Your Vision in Practice

It's essential to have a visual reminder of your vision, so vividness is critical. It's better to have that image somewhere elsewhere, like your idea could be held by your bed and your technical view somewhere at the workplace entrance or right above your head. This way, you can check up and refer to it regularly.

Keeping it noticeable can help you stay on track by offering advice as opportunities or distractions occur. When you can see that dream clearly, you can always doubt how your current actions lead to that ultimate goal.

Ask yourself with every new day: if this was my last day to work towards my ultimate goal, would I spend it this way?

Personal Vision

Your vision directs you in your everyday life as you set goals and have to make decisions. Reflect on different perspectives when developing your vision, and talk about what you want to get, be, give, and do.

How can you add to this environment, affect your inner circle, your society, or even people on this planet and support them? Thinking about that also exposes your real-life intent.

The best way to imagine a personal vision for your future in a vision board.

Organizational Vision

The organizational vision is the core and cornerstone of every corporate strategy, mainly the goals. The dream serves as the "north pole"-it refers to workers' day-to-day jobs as a commitment to the overall long-term accomplishment.

A dream typically presents itself in a mission declaration in businesses or non-profit organizations.

CHAPTER 4: STOPPING TO DOUBT ONES GREATNESS AND WHY WE NEED IT

We all have ambitions that are out of control. Eat healthier. Eat healthier. Exercise more. Exercise more. Lose weight. Lose weight. Head early to home. If we think we want to do, have or accomplish it, it just keeps going; it's not going to happen.

This is the most challenging aspect of human behavior.

It might be anything from startup to writing a book to cook or drawing more. It might be anything. Health and wellness writer Darya Rose refers to it as "I don't like it's a fraud," and talks about how it undermines its culinary activities. Seth Godin calls it "the rebellion." This plagues us all; irrespective of what you choose to request this. Yet this must not be the way!

Here are the steps to go beyond it.

Phase 1: Through the desire to mark oneself, uncertainty about a goal or new behavior is one aspect. But when we have a bad day, it is another to place on a small, pejorative sticker. They say such things like,' I am tired," I am unmotivated," I have no motivation' or, worst of all,' I am unable.' When, though, you settle down for the mark, you compromise your accomplishments and get into a downward spiral of shame and guilt. Resist the need to mark a disappointment yourself and figure out instead why you are dealing with this specific problem.

Phase 2. If you sense your pace slowing down and vitality flickering, ask why. Channel your inner three-year-old. And then ask why —-like a kid (I don't have to tell you how it works if you have one).

Take the classic example: "I don't want to work out." Why? "Why are you tired? Because I'm tired." "Because I work a lot, and I have had difficulty sleeping." Why are you sleeping trouble? "Because I'm under tension." Why? "And I thought I don't have the energy to do what I want to do." All right! We get somewhere now.

Phase 3: Identify the Huge, why you are suddenly trying to figure out why you don't want to train, and where reasons come from. So, let's have a broad look: why would you want to teach first? "I don't like how I look and feel, because I don't like it." "Since I got a couple of pounds, and I feel out of shape." So why do you want to practice? "Why can't you be this person?" "Because I see others exercising, and they seem so fit and energized. "And," — and it's here— "I don't want to get the best out of shape in the school or go through the woods. I'm afraid I can't ever become one of those healthy, good guys." Evidence is clear: our opinions are significant. If we don't feel that we are right or deserving, our inspiration disappears.

Phase 4: Challenge the confidence. Instead of eating your reasons outright, question them. Look at them like you'd have anything about which you're doubtful.

Follow your "why" with "who says?" Who says you can't find time to move your body every week? That said, it must be in the fitness center? Who said you couldn't be happy and fit?

Once you recognize the false belief, you can see it in fear. You realize that anxiety is the first move to overcoming it.

Phase 5: Look past emotions. Well, we all have our days when it doesn't matter whether we write a book or when we sort a laundry. But an emotional response must not govern you. Because feelings disappear, and once they are, you're there again in your life. You deserve the things you most want, of course. And you can't have them for any reason.

Understanding why you do it and that you can do it in a way that works in your life is the secret to developing routines that help your objectives. And when you realize why and why everything begins to change. Just look. Just watch.

4.1 Learning's from Our Worst Conversations

Conversational Intelligence takes the listening skills a step further by offering "listening" with more contexts. Glaser uses the idea of "deconstruction of conversation," which looks back to look forward. Examine a discussion to collect new insights after reality. When we start a conversation, our brain decides if the other person is to trust. If that effect "feels good," we'll be working towards opening up to more experiences. If that impact "feels bad," we're going to close and move into protective mode.

Here are a few questions for exploration and learning in the deconstruction process.

Did anyone addict to being right?

Have you had the Tell-Sell-Yell syndrome? (Tell them once, try selling them why you're right, then yell!) Have you ever asked questions you already knew the answers?

If you said YES to any of these queries, you worked from the primitive brain pumping cortisol (amygdala), holding you in a safe state of mistrust.

So how do you shift from this part of your brain that is triggered by menacing behaviors? The very first step is recognizing the neurological response and finding ways to move away from fears. Understand the root of the worries, work backward to find a solution.

How do we sideline the Amygdala signals?

Note how we respond to threats (fighting, flight, freezing, appeasement) Recognize this reaction Consider if we always choose the same response and how much the danger affects us Choose an alternate way to react at the moment (methods of mindfulness: breathing in, breathing out, voicing how you feel).

4.2 Moving from Distrust to Trust

If we speak to somebody, a lot depends on the attitude of both parties. Is there a level of trust or lack of confidence?

Now, what if you could find such daunting interactions easier to navigate and produce positive, successful results? The reaction is, would you!

But first, there are several lessons to learn about how our brains work to move from mistrust to confidence. Knowing how our minds work with greater ease will contribute to creating safe, trusting relationships.

We see nature in a state of mistrust by terror and intimidation, and we near. We prefer to withdraw, which places us in a state of "defense." Our primitive or reptilian brain is triggered by feeling stressed or threatened. The body releases higher cortisol and adrenaline, so the brain's anxiety networks place us in a condition of run, flight, freeze, or compromise dubbed "Amygdala Hijacking." In Judith Glaser's book "Conversational Intelligence," she explores how confidence in her Truth paradigm shifts our truth. According to Glaser, if we are in a place of distrust we are:

- Interpret with fear

- Interpret with fear

- Interpret with fear

- Tell secrets

- 'Yes' people

If we expect to be in a position to shift to a state of trust, our body releases those' Shifts of thought to the prefrontal cortex (where executive functions reside). It is there that we have exposure to empathy, reasoning, higher decision-making, and imaginative faculties.

Once there, we will calm, create a state of trust, and become accessible to interaction. Glaser spells truth in this "confidence zone" with very different results. We can deal with REALITY in our "confidence state":

- Reveal more

- Expect less and more deliver

- Look with an open heart

- Interpret with facts

- Tell the truth

- Yes, to confront the truth

When we understand how the human brain works, the invisible one. We will potentially retrain the lima bean formed amygdala–the area(s) of our brains that are seen as having a primary function in memory consolidation, emotional reactions, and decision making –to respond more healthily. Then we can switch our interactions from transactional (info-exchange) to transformational (share and discover).

Yeah, remember you have an option every time you're nervous. You can respond with frustration and shut yourself down (where you reside with distrust), or you can choose to calm yourself down and step into a more relaxed, comfortable environment.

As Judith Glaser points out in "Conversational Intelligence: Why Great Leaders Achieve Extraordinary Results":

"To achieve the next stage of grandeur depends on the quality of the society, which depends on the nature of the interactions and depends on the quality of the conversations. It all happens in conversations.

4.3 How to Let Go of Past

All of us were wounded. You cannot be an adult — or adolescent — alive today who hasn't felt any sort of emotional distress.

It does hurt. That's what I get.

But perhaps more important than the hurt itself is what you do with that hurt. Would you instead be returning to being an active life liver? Or do you tend to continually ruminate about the past and something that cannot be changed?

In brief, how do you suffer and pass on from past hurts? Let's find out Blaming our pain on others is what most of us are doing. Anyone did something wrong because, in some sense, they wronged us that mattered to us. We would like to apologize to them. We want them to accept that what they did was wrong.

But, as Holly Brown notes, blaming someone else for our hurt can backfire because it can often leave you powerless. For e.g., you're questioning the individual (your supervisor, partner, parent, child), and they're responding, "No, I didn't," or worse, "What if I did? "You're stuck with all that anger and hurt, and there's no resolution.

Both opinions are valid. It's necessary to experience them truly, and then go on. Nursing your grievances is a bad habit as it hurts you more than it hurts them (as the title goes).

People who hold on to those past hurts often relive the pain in their minds over and over. Sometimes in this pain, in that hurt, in this guilt, a person can even get "stuck."

Ways of letting go of past hurts

The way to accept happiness in your life is to make room for it. If your heart is full of pain and hurt, then how can you be open to something new?

1. Decide to let it go.

Things don't go away themselves. You have to commit to "let it go." If you don't make a conscious choice upfront, you could end up sabotaging your effort to move on from that past hurt.

Taking the conscious decision to let go requires always acknowledging that you have the option to let go. To stop reliving the past pain, stop going through the details of the story in your mind anytime you hear of the other party (after following stage 2 below). For most individuals, this is motivational, realizing that they decide to either hang on to the suffering or lead a future life without it.

2. Share the frustration — and your responsibility.

Show the distress you've been feeling, whether it's specifically to the other party or just taking it out of mind (like offering it to a relative or writing a letter to the other individual in a newspaper). Take it all out of the account straight away. This will help you understand what your hurt is about — correctly.

We don't live in a black-and-white world, even when it often seems like we do. Although you may not have the same responsibility for the feelings you experienced, there may have been a small part of the hurt you are partly responsible for as well. Next time what could you have done differently? Think about whether you are an active participant in your own life or just a survivor without hope? Do you want to let the suffering become your identity? Or are you someone darker and more complex??

3. Stop being the victim and blaming others.

Being the victim feels good— it's like you're on the world's winning team. But do you know what? Most don't care about the world, so you need to get over yourself. Yes, you are something extraordinary. Hey, the feelings matter. But don't equate that "your feelings matter" as "your feelings will outweigh everything else, and nothing else matters." Your feelings are just a part of this great thing we call life, which is all complicated and nuanced. Yet noisy.

You have that option in every moment— to continue feeling bad about the actions of another person or to start feeling affirmative. take responsibility for your happiness and not put that power into another person's hands. Why are you going to let the individual who harmed you— in the past— have that control right here right now?

No amount of logical rumination has ever solved an issue with the partnership. Never Not in the entire past of this nation. And why do you choose to indulge in so much thinking and dedicate so much time to a person you feel you have wronged?

4. Concentrate on the moment— the here and now — and joy.

Now it is time to let go. Let go and stop reviving the past. Stop telling yourself the tale where the narrator— you— is eternally the object of the horrible actions of this other guy. You can't change the things that happened in the past; all you can do is make the best day of your life today. When memories sink into your consciousness (as they are bound to do from time to time), for a moment, acknowledge them. And then gently take yourself right into the present moment. Most people find it easier to do this with a mental prompt, like thinking to themselves, "its ok. That was the past, and now I'm concentrating on my joy and doing it.

"Note, once we clutter our brains — and lives — with hurt feelings, there's little space for anything useful. It's a choice you make to carry on experiencing pain, rather than bringing pleasure back into your life.

5. Forgive them— and you.

We may not have to forget the bad behaviors of another person, but virtually everyone deserves our pardon. Sometimes in our pain and stubbornness, we get stuck; we can't even imagine forgiveness. Yet forgiving doesn't mean, "I approve with what you've done." Instead, it says, "I don't agree with what you've done, yet I forgive you nonetheless." Forgiving isn't a flaw. Instead, it just states, "I'm the right person. You're a good human being. You have done something which hurt me. But in my life, I want to move ahead and welcome joy back into it. I can't do that absolutely before I let go of everything. "Forgiveness is a means to let go of something real. It's also a chance to empathize with the other individual, and to try to see things from their viewpoint.

So, forgiving oneself can also be an essential part of this phase, as we may end up punishing ourselves for the problem or pain at times. While we may have played a role in the pain, there is no justification you need to continue beating yourself over it. If you cannot forgive yourself, how can you live in peace and happiness in the future?

4.4 The Secret to Independence

According to Isa Judd, author of the books Love Has Wings and Why Walk When You Could Fly. "Most of us live in a codependent relationship, with our families, friends, or social group." She said we let others form our beliefs and choices — so much so that we lose sight of who we are.

Darlene Lancer, MFT, psychotherapist and author of Codependency for Dummies, also noted that many people are not fully autonomous, instead "forming our feelings and behaviors about anything external." You write the laws through which you live. This means "owning your reality, your views, your emotions, your feelings, your beliefs [and] memories." Autonomy means having "the confidence that we have in ourselves, our self-awareness to know who we are and what we want," says Judd. I don't trust myself or my actions when I don't embrace myself, and I let other people know who I am and how I act.' Below, Judd and Lancer shared their ideas as to how we can become self-sufficient step by step.

1. Get to know yourself.

"If you do not know who you are, you can't be independent, "said Lancer. She suggested that she think about what happened during your day to get acquainted with yourself.

Ask yourself, "Have I spoken my truth? "Remember the difference between what you feel inside and the words you say to the world and your actions." You can, for example, say yes to something that you don't want to do, said Lancer. What can you know from this?

2. Challenge your biases and convictions.

Observe your convictions, and Judd said he was willing to ask them questions. "Perhaps our views are so normal that we can't stop to see whether they represent what we feel: kneejerk reactions simply reaffirming the past. Also, our outer environments and those around us are influencing those viewpoints. She said that re-evaluating our views of ourselves and the environment is essential to development. There can be no evolution without change."

3. Make yourself assertive.

Assertive will be a powerful way to enhance your life and increase self-confidence, which in turn will help you to become confident, said Lancer.

Efficiency is the ability that you can learn. This means setting healthy boundaries, learning to say no, and understanding your needs and feelings.

It means that you respect yourself and others. According to the psychologist Randy Paterson, Ph. D, we establish communication with ourselves and with others through assertiveness in The Assertiveness Workbook. We become real people with real ideas, real differences, and actual defects. And all this stuff we say. We're not pretending to become another mirror. We don't try to suppress the uniqueness of someone else. We're not trying to pretend we're perfect. We become ourselves. We become ourselves. We're allowed to be there.

4. Start making your own choices.

One way to make your own decisions is to figure out how your day will be, said Lancer. Ask yourself: "I want to do what? "Take your interests and passions into consideration," she said.

5. Comply with your needs.

People in codependent relationships are great to meet the needs of others but generally ignore their own needs, said Lancer. Everyone has different needs, including mental, financial, physical, and spiritual needs.

Lancer said, define your needs and find ways to meet them. For example, if you know that you feel lonely; answer your need by reaching out to a close friend and preparing dinner. "It is becoming autonomous."

6. Learn to calm down.

Acknowledge and express your feelings. As usually said,"' I should not feel that way'" or neglect your emotions, be a good parent, and comfort. Take the time to find what makes you calm and happy.

Also, it means living by "your internal guidance system" instead of external systems, Lancer said. And it's key to accomplishment. "We can never feel satisfied by chasing someone else's dreams: the only way we can find true fulfillment is to live independently.

Chapter 5: THE SECRET OF LIVING WITHOUT EXCUSES

Every day, people wrongly make excuses for the challenges they face. If you can learn to remove 99 percent of your life's reasons, then you can focus your energy on getting results to overcome these challenges.

* Benefits of Eliminating Excuses

* More results

* Less waste of time

* People will appreciate it more

* Great personality benefits

* Lower stress

* Better work ethics

* Learning new skills

Excuses are part of everybody's life. Living 100 percent free of explanation is almost impossible, but with a lot of practice and dedication, you can get very close. Experience as an excuse free as you can release you from the "I can't because" or "I didn't because" negative cycle to place you in a position that allows you to overcome obstacles and challenges. Excuses are subconsciously stopping you from achieving your goals or even trying in some cases. Excuses are made up for several reasons like the inability to do the task, not being prepared, and many other purposes. People have a tendency to make excuses for not having to do anything. The concern is that most of the time, people are going to waste more stressing money and making significant efforts to make up an excuse than the real-time it would have taken to complete the job.

Everyone has time limits. The learning of time management and maximizing wasted time is a great personal development tool. When you're in a workplace environment, the supervisor or clients would greatly appreciate that you're making an effort just to do stuff, rather than excuses. Who would you prefer the mechanic who gets it fixed on your car or the one who keeps telling you why he didn't have it yet?

It will not only support you at work but wherever you go and with whatever you do. There is an opportunity to overcome these challenges and learn new skills by accepting challenges as they are presented. There are difficulties (aka problems) in everybody's life. The disparity in how much tension you are generating from these problems relies on how you handle the situation. When you continually make up excuses and never get performance, you actually do an insult to yourself. The good news is that it can remove obstacles and transform them into a meaningful learning experience. Keep reading, and I'm going to give you some tips and advice to start living without excuses.

Direct you to a Free Life Excuse Know how to find your reasons before you take action think off the Box for Problem Solving Be Able to Understand Challenging & Live Life Excuse Free Start Crashing & Laziness Having an excuse is very helpful in terms of accomplishment. As mentioned earlier, living 100 percent free of reason would be almost impossible, but instead of trying to achieve a goal that is nearly unattainable, try to change as many ideas as you can for results. This won't change overnight, but rather an ongoing process, which will slowly change your behavior, until you come out of your habit of excuse. If you can just find one less argument each day, take faith that your actions will have a significant impact on your life.

Excuses can be a complicated concept to understand in the first place. Many people will end up dismissing their reasons or trying to justify them as "good excuses."

It doesn't care if it's an explanation for its success or not. Begin evaluating the interactions of others or what you talk to yourself in the language of your minds to help identify the reasons. Search for threats or problems that might emerge, and talk about how you want to respond to them. When you continually build excuses, why you can't or won't sit back and consider the root cause of creating the justification. Reasons are literally excusing you give not to do anything. They're locking you out of the champion group.

Some Phrases That Either Lead to Excuses

- If...

- I can't do it because...

- If I had... I could.

- ... has happened to me

- .... It's not fair.

- ... is having an advantage.

Let's explain why that's not possible.

- I'm not getting enough time.

- I don't have the income.

- I don't know how to do it...

It's time to stop them once you've learned what reasons are. Avoid them by either transforming your emotions into more positive and productive ones or doing the opposite step of what you would do if you were to pursue the reasons. Another example will be if you think you can't try anything anyway.

It is surprising to find out that something is better than you initially thought, and you have a chance to actually complete it. Remember, if you're never trying, then you've got a 100% chance of failure.

Traditionally, if you fail on a number of occasions, you will really believe you don't have the skills and knowledge to do that. This is where you'll have to think outside the box in order to challenge your conviction. Excuses are ways we can cope with things that cause us frustration and stress, but they're not helping us grow and learn. If you have failed and given up on something, try to tackle the problem with a different approach rather than making excuses. Take the time to plan your solution, or you might even ask others for advice. Do not do the exact same thing, and expect a different outcome. Make your attempt change; this is the only way you'll ever learn and grow. Consider life's challenges and persevere until you get the desired result. If you begin to face problems and treat them as challenges, your quality of life will significantly improve. You'll probably build a good deal of trust in yourself.

Another significant impediment to us is laziness and procrastination. These two barriers stand out at the top of the list for why people are making excuses and not accepting challenges. Inertia stops us from trying, so we really do not want to get going. When we're caught in the lazy loop our need just to be idle is so strong that we're going to make up excuse after excuse to avoid having to do any real work or even initiate a competition. All you have to do to break the cycle of laziness is actually get going and stay with it. Push aside your excuses and take action now.

The other primary reason people make up reasons is procrastination. Do not wait until your life is dominated by the ideas, take control of them now. As soon as you do, you know how much talent you have and how much more fun you can do. This is an excellent skill for you to learn through personal development on your journey.

5.1 Love the One You Is

For many, the self-love idea might conjure up images of tree-hugging hippies or old self-help books. Yet, as many psychology studies show, the secret to mental health and well-being is self-love and -compassion, holding depression and anxiety at bay.

Cultivating self-love sentiments can be challenging at times.

"Why is it so important to love oneself?" you might ask. Self-love may seem like a luxury instead of a necessity for many of us or new age for those who have too much time in their hands.

Ironically, however, those of us who work too hard and are continually striving to surpass ourselves and grasp the shape-shifting phantasm of perfection might actually need most self-care and compassion.

When we're too hard on ourselves, we do it most of the time because we're driven by a desire to excel by doing everything right all the time. This involves a lot of self-criticisms, and a hallmark of perfectionism is that persecutory inner voice that continually tells us how we could have done things better.

It is concluded that perfectionists are at a higher risk of multiple diseases, both physical and mental, and that self-compassion could liberate us from its grip. Perfectionism and self-compassion are, therefore, inextricably tied together.

The post would explore methods of dialing down the former and improving the latter, with the belief that doing so will help you live a healthier, fuller life.

Most of us in the Western world were raised to believe that perfectionism is of high quality. After all, becoming concerned with precise specifics contributes to great jobs, and this quality of attitude gives us a chance to humble brag during job interviews.

And perfectionism is bad for you, in fact. Not just "not perfect" or "excessively negative" but deliberately evil. As in the case of tobacco or obesity.

A reduced lifetime, irritable bowel syndrome, fibromyalgia, eating disorders, insomnia, and susceptibility to suicide are just a few of the adverse health effects related to perfectionism.

It is also more difficult for perfectionists to recover from heart disease or cancer, which makes both survivors and the general population more susceptible to anxiety and depression.

Out of Perfectionism

So how can we stop Perfectionism? First of all, know this is terrible for you; it slowly smoothest you over every little error and leaves you less satisfied. And something more than that, you deserve.

"Love, connection, and acceptance are your birthright." Kristin Neff, professor of human development of Austin's University of Texas, said. "Bliss is something to which you have the right, not something you need to earn. Paul Hewitt— a clinical psychologist in Vancouver (Canada) and author of the book "Perfectionism: A Relational Approach to Conceptualization, evaluation, and treatment" (Perfectionism: A Relational Approach to Treatment) likes an interior critique harbored by perfectionists to "a nasty adult blowing a small child with the crap."

Perfectionists will continuously give themselves a hard time over the most unexpected things from missing a deadline to dropping a teaspoon on the floor— so criticizing yourself for criticizing yourself isn't uncommon.

Third, you can begin to cultivate some much-needed self-compassion. You may think self-love is a matter of "you either have it or you don't," however, thankfully, researchers maintain that you can acquire it.

What is compassion for oneself? Within technical research, Self-compassion and self-love are commonly used interchangeably.

But what exactly is it? Drawing on Prof. Neff's research, Sabra and colleagues describe self-compassion as a concept that includes three components:

- self-kindness (i.e., treating oneself with empathy and forgiveness),
- appreciation of one's role in a shared humanity (i.e., acceptance that humans are not flawless and specific encounters are part of a more significant human experience),
- And consciousness (i.e., knowledge of one's position in shared humanity); Neff, Gerber.

Are you saying easier than done? You may think so, but fortunately, the same researchers who have worked defined the feeling have also come up with some useful tips for improving it.

Mindfully trained self-compassion

In the researchers ' words,' Self-compassion says,' Be kind to you in the midst of suffering and it will change.' Mindfulness means' Open to suffering from spacious awareness, and it will change." The program includes various meditations, such as' loving-kindness meditation' or' affected breathing' and' informal practices.'

Practicing such techniques for 40 minutes every day for eight weeks, according to the researchers, increased the level of self-compassion of the participants by 43 percent.

There are various exercises in mindfulness that one can do to develop self-compassion. Another simple practice includes saying the following three phrases at moments of emotional distress: "This is a period of pain," "Pain is a part of life," and "Can I be kind to myself." These three mantras refer to the three aspects of self-love we introduced earlier.

Prof. Neff outlines many more valuable mantras in her book Self-Compassion and advises the reader to create their own. Additionally, her self-compassion.org page offers a wide range of similar exercises, which are freely accessible.

When you feel a bit dubious about the effects of actively reinforcing mantras to yourself, you can benefit from knowing they are backed up by the study.

These vigilant self-compassion activities have been shown to lower levels of cortisol stress hormone and improve variation of heart rate, which is the natural capacity of your body to manage stressful situations.

Learning to listen to one another

Listening to one another can mean two things. Firstly, paying attention to how you speak to yourself internally is crucial to learning how to cultivate an intimate sense of self-love.

Writing yourself in a compassionate tone can help.

Throughout their book, Professor NEF encourages her students to question themselves, "That kind of vocabulary do you use with yourself if you find a fault or make a mistake? Do you blame yourself or choose a tone of more forgiving and understanding? How do you act inside of yourself, if you are extremely self-critical? "So, to replace this loud inner voice with a kinder one, you can just notice it— which is already a step towards quietly subduing it— and try to soften it actively.

Finally, in the language of a kinder, more compassionate soul, you should attempt to rephrase the conclusions you may have articulated initially very harshly.

Or, from the perspective of the kind, compassionate friend you've been to others, or from the perspective of a sympathetic friend, you could try writing a letter to yourself.

A second reason why listening is relevant, is that you can prove invaluable during periods of emotional distress by asking yourself the question "What do I need?" — And listening attentively to the answer.

As scholars point out, "Just asking the question is itself an exercise in self-compassion— fostering goodwill towards oneself." But it's also worth considering in mind that "What do I need?" often implies that an emotionally distressed person will avoid meditating entirely and react behaviorally to his or her emotional distress, e.g., by drinking a cup of tea

Yoga and relearning pleasure

Knowledge may help us relearn, as adults, to appreciate simple, everyday things we used to enjoy spontaneously as kids. Reconnecting ourselves in this way with pleasure is an essential component of self-kindness. Such techniques are intimately linked to the habit of listening to yourself and to your needs.

Maybe because yoga will help us get back in touch with our own bodies and recover a sense of pleasure from it, the activity always tends to silence our inner critic's voice and raise self-love sentiments.

Try to enjoy the process as you pass through it; perhaps one day, you can realize that the nagging sense of incompleteness that is so characteristic of perfectionism has left you.

Instead, you'll have cultivated a more childish, self-forgiving sense of wholeness.

5.2 Being from Where You Are

Just imagine how liberating it would be!

Any move we make in our teens and twenties is motivated by the opinions of other people. And as we age, if we move in the right direction, our obsession with how others perceive us begins to trickle away, but very few of us are capable of completely escape its pointless grasp.

In the meantime, the fact is, the only issues you'll ever have to answer while making life choices are:

1. Is this something I want, do, or do I want to be?

2. Will this lead me in the way I want to (shouldn't) go?

3. Will that screw someone else over* in the process?

When we live in fear of others, we throw a wet blanket of ho-hummers over our lives, instead of celebrating who we are.

Sure, caring is part of our survival instinct — get kicked from the group, and you'll be freezing to death or starving or being eaten by wolves. But since we have big brains and the power to manifest anything to which we set our minds, there is another story that is equally plausible: get booted from the tribe and create, or discover, another tribe that is more of your type. Not only could you wind up doing what you do surround by people you love with whom you actually relate, but one day you might find that you can no longer remember the names of those people whose recognition you once badly felt you would suffer without.

No one who has ever accomplished anything significant or new or worth raising a celebratory fist in the air has done so from their comfort zone. They risked ridicule and failure, and even death on occasion. Think about brothers Wright. Can you imagine how it all went down?

When you step away from the crowd and let your true self show, you are likely to find yourself in front of the perception firing squad (especially if what you want to do is exceptional and beyond the comfort zones of everyone), which is why so many people are screaming out of their life that they would love to live. It's a gamble, only enabling you to be seen. Look at how we treat celebrities — their every move is picked up and passed on, discussed, judged, and photographed without making up. It is astonishing that only half of them spend time in rehab.

You're in charge of what you say and do. You are not responsible for whether people freak out on it or not. Assume Two people walking out of the same show, one person sticking to the doors, bloodshot and distraught, leaving a trail of tears, more shaken by this film than any other movie in cinema history, while the other person walks up to the ticket counter and demands money back because she felt it was the worst piece of garbage ever to be shown.

One motion picture, two very different experiences. Why? For what? It's about the moviegoers because it's not about the movie. The trick is not only to deny any power over you to criticize but, even more challenging. There's nothing wrong with accepting a compliment blushingly, but if you're always looking for outside approval that you're good enough or fresh enough or talented or worthy enough. If you base your self-worth on what everybody else thinks of you, you hand over all your power to other people for validation and become dependent on a source outside yourself.

Then you wind up chasing after something that you have no control over, and you end up with a full-blown identity crisis if something suddenly puts its focus elsewhere, or changes its mind and decides that you are no longer very interesting.

All that matters is what's right for you, and you'll be a mighty superhero if you can stay connected to that without straying.

All else is just the perception of reality by other people, and that is not your business.

So how can't you really worry about what others think and be your most strong self?

1. ASK YOURSELF WHY

Why are you going to say something or do something? Is it likable? Why put down someone, if you feel insecure? To get somebody back because they were making a fat joke about your mom? Or does it come from a realm of strength and truth? Do you do it, because it's going to be fun? Do you feel called to do that, because? Because it will change the life of another in a positive, martyr-free way? Pay attention (be honest), to your motives. Practice this comes from a place of honesty, and you're going to win.

2. ALWAYS DO YOUR BEST

There's no faster way to fall victim to feedback outside than when you feel vulnerable. And there is no better way to feel insecure than to know that you are half-assured of something or that you really does not believe in what you are doing. Regardless of what it is— raising your prices or raising your kids — if you do the absolute best you can and come from a place of integrity, be proud of yourself despite thinking of others.

3. TRUST the INTUITION

Birds use their instincts to fly halfway around the globe to breeding grounds. Deer and rabbits and other beasts of the prey type use their abilities to discourage predators from rushing in. On the other hand, the average human will take their drunk-before-noon neighbor's advice across the street instead of doing what is best deep down, we know. How many times in the hindsight did you think I knew I should have listened to my gut!?

You have an incredible, in-house guidance tool to use whenever you need it. Say that everyone should shut up and go away, get quiet, give themselves room to feel, and think. Inside, you have all the answers. Practice sharpening your intuition by taking the time to strengthen your Source Energy connection, and trust for sure you know what's best. The more centered you are, the stronger you will be (look in this book for more tips on how to do that later).

4. SEEK A TEMPORARY MODEL

Seek a guide or a role model. Make clear why this person is impressive and inspiring to you, and ask yourself, what would my hero do when faced with a challenge that leaves you guessing how to react?

Not caring about what others think is a point that takes some time meanwhile uses this trick while you're still getting healthy, and before you know it, you're going to be able to dissolve your hero and ask yourself what I'd do.

5. LOVE YOURSELF

No matter what others say? While you are not allowed to base your self-worth on what other people think, this does not mean that you should miss the opportunity to benefit from outside input fully.

Input, especially from those who know you well.

There's something like a constructive critique and constructive complementation. But it depends on you whether they are useful, or not.

Suppose if people have been telling you for years that you're a hothead that they feel they can't be open with you because you're blowing up in their faces the second you disagree with them, ask yourself Is this true (be honest)? Can we use this information to improve ourselves and others' lives? If the answer is yes, agree to make the necessary modifications; if the answer is no, let go.

The same is true of compliments. If you're a good listener continually being told by people, ask yourself, is this compliment genuine for me? Can we use this information to improve ourselves and others' lives? Again, if yes is the answer, figure out how you can capitalize on it; if no is the answer, let it go.

Sometimes seeing what we cannot see ourselves is more comfortable for other people, so if it helps us connect with our truths and live a happier, more authentic life, then it's worth taking the time to listen.

Ultimately, though, it still comes down to what's right for you, so the more connected you are to your inner truth, the easier it will be to take advantage of outside opinions, rather than let them govern your life.

The definition of screwing someone over is to take their money and do a poor job or destroy their water source or enslaves populations, things like that— your mother is disappointed, or your father disapproves of it, or your friends are outraged...

5.3 What Are You Doing Here?

The big question is if you'll be able to say a full yes to your adventure.

—Joseph Campbell

American mythologist whose book ideas inspired the creation of Star Wars The distinction between living a happy, fulfilled life of plenty, freedom and expansiveness, or living in a restricting veal pen, of your indecision and tired old excuses, can be obvious about what your real intention is.

A gift is which is obviously meant to be given, that's why it's so brutal when we can't figure out what is ours, or when we know what it is,

 but we're too lame to act. Here is the perfect gift to share with the world, just bursting to be opened, and we keep it sitting there, tightly wrapped in a box, growing old and gathering dust. Oh, rubbish! Agony! An agony!

Meanwhile, there's unparalleled joy in giving someone the perfect gift. We also know how it feels, jumping back and forth from foot to foot, wringing paws, peeing in our socks, practically begging them to unlock it. IT ALREADY OPENS!

Christ Jesus. Let me freak in do it right here! The influence of sharing is so powerful that joy and good feelings are often stronger for the giver than for the recipient. That's why you sound like a rock star as you discover your calling and plan your life so that you can regularly share your talents with the world.

We are in harmony with our best, most strong self, as we express what we were brought here to offer.

However, most people wander through their lives, giving their gifts a tasteful version of the candle. You know— they don't show up to the party empty-handed or anything; they present to the world their somewhat flaccid gift, receive a warm hug, and in return, "Oh, you shouldn't have," but they're not knocking it out of the park. For instance, they get a job doing something they either hate or it's a bit of a yawn, but that's okay, you know. It gives them a life that covers the basics, as long as they are not going too crazy.

They are doing fun things but not as much as they would like because they don't have the resources. Or the pacing. Or the trust which they merit. We have little wins here and there, we hit their sales quota, and they earn the six-day trip to the Caribbean, or they rack up enough miles to live with their aunt and see the Games or finally sit down and write a whole album they may or may not ever produce or sing, but they never really go for it and create a life that really lights them up. We basically give away their lives to Big Snooze.

Every single person is born with talents that are rare and important to share with the world. When we find out what is ours, and decide to live our lives putting them to use, that's when the real party starts, and only then. Everybody has access to living a life on purpose. So, if you're struggling or settling or being totally confused about what you're supposed to do with your life, you know the answer is here already. There is, and so does the experience that you can't wait to create. You just have to get a little clarification first.

Remember that there is no right way to go about this. Everyone's journey is unique and we all are trying to get to the same place — the place we feel the happiest, the most alive, and the one we like.

Even if you've nailed yourself to the perfect career, read on, as these tips can help you in all areas of your life.

How to decide who you are and what your name is:

1. BE THE Astronaut

Think you're an astronaut floating in outer space, and you're unexpectedly swooping down to Earth and living in your own body. As the alien, it's all new to you about this life. You're looking around-what, are you seeing? What's that guy you've inhabited so obviously awesome at? What are they doing the most amusing? What are their connections? What resources and chances are there for them?

As the outsider to whom it's all new and exciting and there's nothing at stake and no history to drag around, what are you supposed to do with this fantastic new existence you've entered? How will you use this new body and this existence to start creating something fabulous and awesome right now?

This technique is of tremendous help to get a new perspective and get beyond our boring-ass ruts with tired old explanations and weak routines

. It can also be instrumental in making you aware of all the astounding possibilities and resources you have at your fingertips and don't see. Sometimes looking at things with new eyes is as simple as understanding how astonishingly fortunate we are. Be the twenty-four-hour alien, and know what you are coming up with.

2. TAKE THE FIRST RIGHT STEP

Instead of wasting hours figuring out your next perfect move, just already do something. Oh, the time we spend rolling ideas in our heads, imagining what-ifs, coming up with excellent reasons why they are perfect and why not perfect reasons, tearing at our cuticles, making our friends and family screen their calls carefully in case it's us again, wanting to go over some ideas. Get out of your mind, and do something. You don't have to know precisely where it's going to take you, you just have to start with one thing that feels right and then be determined to keep following things and see where they're leading.

It was ironically in the midst of a lifelong obsession with figuring out what the hell was my purpose, when we discovered people being called as a coach. Although it is also understood that writing is part of it, wave always realized that we are not supposed to spend our life in a silent room alone, fighting words into submission. We need something that

A) Included engaging with other people

B) Helped people in some sort of straightforward way

C) was really enjoyable and

D) Require to bathe, dress, and quit. That's all we have to go on with, that the intense desire to figure out.

No matter what you feel right now, keep an eye on suggestions and opportunities that suddenly come up.

So, remember how you think is there something for you that sound like it might be useful to check out, for whatever reason? What did you say you would love to do forever? Has anyone discussed a course or tutor, or a book that remains in your mind? Take the first step toward something that feels right, and see where it's leading you. And NOW do it.

3. DO YOUR BEST WHEREVER YOU'RE AT

When you take this first step, you may not land straight away in your ideal scenario. You could land on a stepping-pitch. It might be a fantastic stepping-stone, or it might be an unpleasant stepping-stone. So irrespective of where your first move takes you, if you want to keep moving ahead, enjoy wherever you are, rather than feeling ashamed or grouchy or anxious. Everything that you do along the way contributes to where you go.

Let's presume you've wanted to go after your dream of being a rock star, and you're taking a job waiting tables so you can fly and play gigs and go to the studio with the freedom. Obviously, your calling is playing music, not caring that the French onion soup of some whiney consumer is supposedly too cold, but it's crucial you matter anyway. Having a good outlook and being thankful for all the things that help you live the life of dreams will not only make life a more enjoyable place to be, and give you more significant tips, but it will also increase your level and draw the people and resources that will carry you in the path you desire.

This is where it always comes in handy to be present in the moment. You may not be on stage in front of thousands doing a split in the air, but remember that you're going for it, you're moving bravely toward your dream, and you're surrounded by incredible miracles and possibilities. Lean back and be grateful that you're living on purpose, that you're hanging out at a high frequency, and that all you need is zooming in towards you.

4. DON'T REINVENT THE WHEEL

 Check about, seeing what other people are doing out there. Whose life makes you utterly jealous? What stuff do people do you would love to do too? You don't need to invent from scratch your ideal life, just to figure out what makes you feel alive. So, if it sparks your interest in what someone else is doing, notice. It might mean your call has something in common with theirs.

Get concrete about the things that turn you on in their lives. Is it because they are having to travel around the world? Is it because they have routine that is solid? Is it because they don't have method? Is it they are operating alone? That they are employed in the nude? That they get to be all day outside? That they're working with his hands? Its eyes? Its ears? Their dogs? You're Spouse? The more descriptive that you get; the simpler it is to create an image of what you want.

Read magazines that you're involved in, talk to as many individuals as you can, hang out in places where people hang out to discuss their passions. Put yourself there and you never know what you might learn to inform your next move, or whom you might meet to present your next chance.

5. DON'T GET CAUGHT UP

I think one of the most paralyzing misunderstandings is that we are all meant to have one true calling which comes to us in a powerful flash of soul-defining wisdom. While there are those people who have always known exactly what they want to do, there's a heck of many more of us out there who are wasting most of our days, if not all of our lives, running around searching for who we are under rocks and behind trees.

If you don't have that one, huge, perfect thing you know you've come here to do (the same goes with seeking the one, large, ideal soul mate, BTW),

 let yourself be off the hook and feel good about the reality that you'll actually meet many callings in your lifespan (and likely relationships).

If you think about it, evolving as you age is more sensible anyway. When I think of who I was in my 20s compared to who I am now, I can't imagine anything more unattractive than going after some of the things that resonated with me back then.

Follow what feels right at the moment, every moment, and it's going to lead you through a very extraordinary life.

6. KNOW YOURSELF

If you actually want to get in touch with who you are, what you want to do, and who you want to do that, devotes your time to your intuition.

One of the best ways is to breathe for you for five minutes each day. We spend our time physically and mentally moving ahead at full speed, and literally bulldozing about the very answers we seek because we cannot hear about the din. When you settle down and ask politely, you will receive an answer. Finally, Ultimately. Keep on, remain patient and wait for your inner feedback to learn. You have all the answers; you just have to give them the chance to get through.

7. FOLLOW YOUR FANTASIES

it is suggested something you will probably not like so much, since given you all the kinder, more gentle ways to figure out yourself:

Go into the deep and follow your imagination. What are you fantasizing about when you look out of the windshield of a train, right before you sleep at night, or listen to someone chatting your ear really awkwardly? Do you play stand-up comedy in front of thousands of hysterical fans? Are you ever in the best and most comfortable home surrounded by your beautiful children?

Are you praised all over the world for establishing orphanages? Do this as though money hadn't been an issue. Tap what brings you great joy, not what you think you have to do to survive.

Your visions are the most transparent peepholes we are and what we consider to be incredible. Regardless matter how ridiculous and nonsensical it may seem, they mean something to us and usually represent our strongest and most important depictions. In a universe of loopholes, our dreams are our truths.

In the meantime, if anyone would read our minds and catch us, we would all be mortified it's totally stupid but someone does it, so why can't you? Most of the times, we pretend that we don't know what our call is if we're really horrified to face it because it seems too big or impossible for us to live with it or not.

So, what if you had the audaciousness to put behind your regrets, and the embarrassment because you decided to be gigantic and beautiful and you really did it? What if you decide to do the most exciting thing you've ever thought of, no matter what someone thinks, including your frightened self?

THAT's real.

8. LOVE YOURSELF

Like you are the only one that you have.

5.4 Lead with Your Crotch

There are many options in the head of the beginner but there are few in the experts.

—Sundry Suzuki; Japanese Zen priest, philosopher, instructor often lovingly known as the "Crooked Cucumber" the significant saying is

"Youth is wasted on young people," but It is generally believed that, in some ways anyway, we've still got it occurring in our late teens and early 20s.

Apart from all the anxiety and drama and police escorts home, we still have our little kid-like ability to create "just because" that is still firmly intact, but we also have that newly-hatched adult ability to make tremendous things happen.

Add to this the fact that we are not yet jaded by a long list of failures, and are still under the impression that death is something that happens to other people, we, if you're anything like me, slip into our lives when we're young with an idiotic, yet impressive, disregard for "what-if." Admittedly, remember doing things in the danger department that still have sleeping with light on.

But recall plunging with the same careless oblivion into creative pursuits and, as a result, having completely amazing and thrilling outcomes.

That's why it is considered to hear people say, "If I realized then what I do now, I'm not positive I'd have done anything." Ok, thank goodness, you didn't know if that's a lame-o mentality. You would sit next to a pile of empty beer cans, whining about how you missed your dreams, if you did!

The dilemma is that once we're older and "wiser," often people trade for more "grown-up" representations of life that vary from pure passable to full-on sucking to living entirely in their intent.

They have bought into this idea that being responsible= no longer having fun, that waking up feeling excited about life is for the youth and once we're older, we have to trade that in, settle down and be "realistic."

Do not think about being an insensitive ass or doing the same things we did when we were younger but talking about living our goals always, no matter what stage of life we're in, rather than settling for mediocrity because we don't think anything else is accessible or acceptable. Only for a limited time do we get to be in our bodies, why not celebrate the journey instead of just riding it out until it is over?

We are still allowed to dream, and our desires are always open to us, but as we move through life, we will make the deliberate effort to overcome any prejudices we have, and knock all our doubts from past experiences in the butt, and engage in our own badassery. Whatever it looks to us like. Instead of the list of negatives we have collected over time, we need to focus on the positive, and keep that focus regardless of what flies in our face. And one of the things to do that is to bond with the kid inside. We know how unacceptable that may sound dorky, but just stay here.

Even though you're most definitely turned on by things different than what you were as a teenager today, you can still learn a lot from how you went through living in the old days. And think back: Was there ever a moment in your rhythm, when you felt utter? Where did you create and do things just because it was fun, without worrying about the result? Where couldn't you wait to wake up and go do your situation in the morning? This could signify anything from when you were a little kid running around with a maxi pad sticking to your eye pretending to be a high school pirate,

When you voted Class Clown to always bribe your way past the ladies in the front office to make false announcements about the loud speaker you learned to play guitar while looking at your hands that summer. How have you been most triggered by existence (and if you still feel this way, stay tuned......) and what can you gain from these experiences?

For example, when the singer-guitarist in a band called Crotch one of the most exciting and on-purpose times of life they use the terms "singer," "guitarist," and "band," all very loosely because those at Crotch aren't concerned with things like learning to play instruments or practicing or any of that snooty musicianship crap. They have bigger fish to fry, like talking about our band in loud voices and checking out in plate glass windows as we walked along with guitars tied to our backs.

If you've known what it's to be in your groove and have trouble finding your way right now, think back what your priorities were when you've been fully enlightened about life, and use them to help you get the clarity and kick you need now in the back end. Here are some nuggets of insight I have gleaned from the days of Crotch which I still find useful:

1. WHAT YOU CAN GET AWAY WITH

Life is r-i-d-i-c-u-l-o-u-s. It's so dangerous— we don't have any freakin ' idea of what we're even spinning around here on this globe in the middle of this solar system with who-the-hell-knows-what's beyond it. It absurd to make a big fat deal out of anything. It makes more sense to approach existence with a feeling of, "Why not? "And not a furrowed brow. One of the best things ever done is to make motto "I just want to see what I can get away with. "It takes off all the pressure, puts in the attitude of punk rock and reminds me that life is just a game.

Yes, we have more significant responsibilities and more pressure as adults, but come on folks; it is guaranteed you there are countless people with way more to whine about out there than you who are totally kicking ass because they decided to go for it instead of sitting around in the wet pant load of their own excuses. Take a new approach to what you are doing and try this on

I just want to see if I can start my own successful business; I just want to know if I can get myself out of debt and make a hundred thousand dollars more this year

Get off the pressure and get back into the adventure.

2. LOSE TRACK OF TIME

Have you ever done something and realized suddenly that hours have passed without you noticing? What's this up for you? And how often that happens during your day? You've officially entered the Vortex when you're so lost in what you're doing that you're losing all sense of time. You want as much as you can achieve hence take a look at your life and figure out how you can make that happen.

Next, find out the stuff in your business and personal life that you get behind. Then figure out how more of the time you can do more of those things. Hire someone (no excuses) and delegate those tasks that you hate to do. Partner with someone who's good at it, and enjoy doing things that you're not in, so you can be released to do more of what you want. If you need to, make massive changes to your business and personal life that will include more time doing what you love. Only work it out. Don't just give up your experience to situations like a little weskit your life take it wherever you desire, so grab it through its nether regions and make it a priority to do the things you love.

3. KEEP BEING THE BEGINNER

When you have no idea how to play your guitar, one of the best things about forming a band is that you don't matter if you suck because you already realize you're doing it. Instead, after you learn how to play, you become all grim, you become overly critical and harsh on yourself, and you no longer let yourself have almost as much fun. The trick is to make the Beginner live alongside the Expert,

 rather than pretending that you don't know who she is when she tries to sit down in the cafeteria with you and your new, more relaxed, more experienced friends. The Beginner might be an idiot, but she knows how to party, and if you don't let her play with you anymore, there's a risk of things getting drilling around. So, refine your skills; take your art seriously; know what you need to do; believe in yourself; work your butt off; fall off; get up; keep going; get really good at what you're doing, but don't forget the joy in that process. Because then, hey, what is the meaning of doing all that work? The only thing you need is get the most out of it. The only other thing that matters once you've achieved that is that you like yourself.

4. LOVE YOURSELF

And your eternal backup singers will be the bluebirds of joy.

CHAPTER 6: EMBRACE YOUR QUEST FOR LIFE

Ancient Greece can be traced back to the idea of living to the utmost by hanging on to life and keeping on close. Research conducted by me and colleagues on the forms in which Greeks, from ancient times to the present day, celebrate the fullness of life along the road of meaning can be seen as an example of how reality is art and how art, in effect, will transform into existence. For example, Greek design commonly known as the "Greek Key." Typically, we see this ornamental pattern, consisting of repeated, continuous vertical and horizontal lines, used artistically as a decorative border on buildings and other artifacts.

In ancient Greece, the Greek key has deep roots. In ancient times this decorative element was called a meander, or meandrous, and had a profound meaning. The term "meander" came to apply to the Maeander River (also spelled Meander) twisting and turning road, which is in what is now southwestern Turkey. Meander has also been used since to define a winding pattern or style.

It has taken on new definitions and uses over time, implying that meander are equivalent to wandering aimlessly and idly, without any set intent or path. Therefore, we now hear common phrases, such as "meandering through life," to describe a form of goalless wandering that is deemed to have no authentic meaning.

The exact origin, interpretation, and use of the Greek key, or meandrous, have been locked away for some 2,500 years. The significance of the ancient Greek meandrous has finally seen the light of day thanks to the groundbreaking research in modern Greece.

In this respect, a Greek expert in the history of religion, Michael Kilojoules, noticed that the meandrous was not meant to be solely a decorative emblem for use in sculpture. On the contrary, the meandrous ' historical and mythological roots indicated that it was a unique handgrip used in ancient Greek gymnastics, in the "pan ration," a Greek martial art which was a popular event at the earliest Olympic Games; and in combat.

Source: Global Language Institute, used with permission According to Kilojoules, on a physical plane, the meandrous grip was the unique joining of hands that was an effective way to secure combatants. The meandrous embrace was a reflection of the noble and enduring Greek spirit on a much larger, spiritual dimension. In metaphorical words, it enabled ancient Greeks to defy the gods. The sign of the meandrous was a confirmation that people, literally and figuratively, kept in their hearts the ability to face with courage whatever happened to come their way in life.

Article goes on after advertising against the most daunting challenges, both internally and externally, the meandrous told the Greeks that they and none other hold the keys to their ultimate destiny. Relying on the hold of the meandrous often implied that they had a purpose in life and were therefore not "meandering" through life or wandering aimlessly, as the word is generally (miss)understood to imply to this very day.

The second source of insight on the Greek key emerged from what seemed to be an unlikely source at first. A famous Greek musician, Gianni's Millikan, has taken leave of the music to research the meandrous ' roots. He published a book, Meandrous: The Forgotten Ancient Greek Gymnastics, in 2010. In it, Millikan defines the meandrous hold, in a similar fashion to Kilojoules, both as a tool for subduing and capturing enemies of different kinds and as a sign of human capacity to overcome adversity no matter how high the odds may be.

Moreover, both Millikan and Kilojoules noticed that even the renowned ancient Greek philosopher Plato, who was an ardent wrestler, was mindful of the grasp of the meandrous. Millikan goes further by implying that the grip of the meandrous symbolizes harmony and power within one's being and in meaningful connections with others. He also reveals the many health benefits that come from exercising the meandrous grip in all areas of life in body, mind and spirit.

The Greek key's true meaning, or meandrous, tells us to hold on life and live it to the fullest. Viewed in this sense, the commonly heard saying, "get a grip," takes an entirely different meaning, one that is simultaneously optimistic and encouraging, by asking us to accept all of life— both ups and downs, joys and sorrows — not merely to tiptoe or walk through it aimlessly.

6.1 How to conquer any challenge

If things go your way, it's easy to feel optimistic but do you contact overwhelmed as soon as problems arise?

When you encounter unforeseen obstacles, it can be hard to keep plugging in, but maintaining your attitude and working on your target will help you stay motivated and benefit from the problem you face.

Developing strategies to tackle and overcome these challenges is all part of a precious life journey.

When you feel disempowered and find it challenging to deal with an obstacle in your life, taking in some time in planning and seeking out a new response to hardship is worthwhile. Having an action plan to deal with stressful situations can help, so here's a few ways to keep smiling, even during those rainy days!

Use these five healthy ideas when faced with a challenge.

1. Center your attention.

Brain is a compelling thing and a healthy way to bring it into your existence is to center on something.

Focusing on the downside, or the barrier to your progress, will expand the issue and keep you from going forward.

Registered Racing Drivers are shown how to concentrate on where their vehicle needs to go. When they focus on the target, they're much more likely to hit it, but they have a much higher chance of success when concentrating on the aim.

Create an image of yourself in the middle of your mind that overcomes the struggle. How do you feel? Reflect on this sensation and it's going to become part of your dream, offering you the power to do it.

2. Earn what you can, wherever you are.

Facing a head-on challenge can be overwhelming. If it seems insurmountable what you are doing, it can be tempting to see yourself as a loser and to give up without really trying to overcome the obstacle.

Starting where you are and making small steps in the right direction will lead you gradually to your goal before you know you've accomplished it little by little. Mountains aren't all scaled at once, after all, but by a series of small moves!

3. Believe in Yourself.

A bit of self-confidence can go a really long way?

It will only be possible to reach your goal if you truly believe you can do it, so take inspiration from those around you when you're flagging.

If somebody asks you, they can do this, believe them! Hear them, let their belief in you strengthen your self-confidence, and you are well on the way to success.

Affirmations can be a handy tool, but set your expectations high and don't let the self-doubt drag you down!

4. Separate yourself from the challenge.

If you face adversity, it can be hard to keep on feeling positive for yourself; if things don't go our way; we always try to analyze the scenario to see where we're going wrong and end up blaming ourselves for it.

It can help to realize that the difficulty that lies ahead is not a sign of who you are: this struggle does not describe you.

That viewpoint will allow you to detach yourself from the task, which can motivate you to progress through it.

5. Don't quit... even if you don't succeed.

The challenges are difficult to overcome by their very nature. If it were not tough it would not be a challenge!

Many days, we can believe we are never going to meet the challenge ahead of us, and it may seem better to give up and hide under the coverings. But we should never allow ourselves to quit, even if it takes longer than we thought at first.

Progress means we get somewhere, even though it's just a little bit at a time. So, step on, also very gradually, means you've done everything–you're better off than before.

And, note every time you're met with a task, a positive approach can really turn things around for you and make it much more likely to succeed.

6.2 The Road to Self-Knowledge

Self-awareness is an ability that anyone with the correct activities and routines will develop and enhance.

Are there parts of your life that you simply couldn't understand? Perhaps there are growing habits or patterns that seem to pop up again and again despite leading to negative results?

The willingness to be self-conscious is one of the most critical and challenging qualities we humans can acquire. But it can be!

In this guide, I'll explain what self-consciousness is, why it's essential, and then walk through 10 useful and practical exercises you can use actually to cultivate self-awareness in your life.

What is Self-consciousness?

Self-awareness involves becoming used to paying attention to the way you perceive, behave and conduct.

• That means looking for trends in the way we tend to think about and interpret what's going on, how we explain things to ourselves, and how we make sense of the world around us.

• It's about knowing our own thoughts and moods. Instead of trying to avoid or "correct" our emotions, we reflect and stay informed about our feelings, even the difficult ones, which are unpleasant.

• In some situations, it means paying attention to how we tend to act and behave. What are our default responses? What are our attitudes and our habits?

In brief, self-awareness involves paying attention to our own personality, and trying to learn it.

How to raise self-confidence

1. Pay attention

To what upsets you about other people often the things that most upset us in other people reflect some quality that we dislike in ourselves.

We all have parts of us which we do not like — a propensity, for example, to bend the truth a little too often. Or perhaps we avoid conflicts such as the flu, sometimes ending up looking like a doormat or becoming exploited by those around us.

If we don't know how to change these things — or believe it's possible — we can end up doing the next best thing: don't think of them. And while indifference can seem like paradise, it really is not. Long-term, not.

So, whenever someone does something that irritates you in particular, ask yourself: Could it be a reflection of something I dislike in me? Is there any variation of that I do?

2. Meditate on your subconscious

You probably heard of meditation on mindfulness. It's the natural process of focusing your attention on your pulse, or some other feeling in physics. Then, if you notice your mind wandering towards other thoughts, gently bringing your attention back to your focus point.

While mindfulness meditation has shown to be beneficial to everything from weight loss to relief from depression, it can be a powerful way to increase your self-awareness level.

In particular, meditation on the mindfulness is one of the best ways to learn more about how your thoughts work. You begin to realize a powerful idea as you learn to follow and analyze our emotions without clinging to them or worrying about them: You are not the feelings.

All too often we lack self-awareness, because we overthink about it. We quickly get lost in our emotions, just because our imagination decided to throw them at us, believing they're real or worth engaging with.

A regular practice in mindfulness will open your eyes to how the mind of consciousness functions and how much more there is than the pure substance of your thinking.

3. Write high quality writing

Good authors are often said to be right critics of the universe around them. And it is this capacity to note subtle details and aspects of life that help them to replicate it in their work so movingly.

But the very best writers in particular are expert observers of human nature. It is their task to note the tiny details of thought, feeling, motivation, and behavior that most of us are lacking in the everyday frenzied business.

And while most of us are indeed not labeled formally to be writers so astute analysts of human nature, we can all learn something or two about ourselves through trying to pay attention like an author.

Through correctly portraying people good writing shows us how to think carefully and compassionately about others. And the better we get in observing others, the more likely we are to look the same way at ourselves.

So sometime spend 30 minutes and come up with a list of good fiction you were reading or telling a smart buddy to pick a few of their favorites.

4. Identify the mental kryptonite

No one likes to feel depressed, nervous, embarrassed or any other negative emotional type. Which is reasonable because they feel inadequate, painfully sometimes so.

And while we all withdraw from negative emotions, every one of us appears to have a single negative feeling that we particularly dislike so try to avoid.

A typical pattern is seen in clinical practice is that patients do whatever they want to avoid feeling depressed. They are going to go to extraordinary— sometimes harmful — lengths to distract or numb that particular feeling of sadness

, even if it means increasing the intensity of other negative emotions such as anxiety, shame, and guilt.

For starters, a client who learned that part of the reason she felt anxious about social situations is that she was always worried that people were criticizing her. Specifically, she was concerned they could tell her that she was drinking too much and was judging her for that.

As asked her about her drinking, we eventually discovered that although alcohol triggered her great deal of embarrassment and fear, it was worth it to her because it was the only way she understood how to escape from the pain of her life.

We all have certain emotions which we particularly dislike. And more often than not, it means we are working really hard not to feel the feeling. The trouble is, being so afraid of an emotion we're able to do just about anything to stop it can contribute to some pretty negative long-term consequences (substance abuse, for example).

But perhaps most notably, we avoid listening to what the feeling has to convey to us, while suppressing the emotion. Negative emotions are unpleasant when our ego, for some excellent reason, is attempting to get our focus.

Learning to tolerate the discomfort of our emotions if we are willing to listen, can unlock a wealth of insight about ourselves.

5. Create a history of your experience

One of the most eye-opening "tricks" is do as a professional also happens with clients during the second session.

Sometimes spend 20 minutes drawing a timeline of their lives at some point before our next meeting, at the end of our first meeting. Sit down with empty sheet of paper and a pencil, and identify the significant events along the continuum of their existence, beginning from their conception.

 Specifically, activities that affected them greatly— big or small, positive or negative.

Inevitably, people come back and say a version of the same thing: it seemed like the stupidest workout ever had, but being surprised at how much you knew.

In fact, by seeing the particular period "in depth" often people can make sense of or get a new perspective on a very distressing or painful time. Being able to think in a cognitive and meaningful manner is crucial to self-awareness.

6. Ask for feedback (and handle it well)

Here's a question: how often do you get input on yourself deliberately? If you are anything like you suspect most people probably not often. Which is a shameful because good feedback is one of the best and most effective ways of developing and improving?

While there are many facets of us that we can see require change, it is the pieces of us that we are unable to recognize — our blind spots — that is the real problem. And others are unique in their position to notice these and help us see them. When we inquire... So how precisely will we ask for feedback about ourselves?

Here are a couple of suggestions;

Choose a stable relationship in your life:

Parent, spouse, best friend... Anyone you have enough respect for a friendship with that they would be willing to point anything terrible out.

Limited company.

First talk about something that isn't too large or dangerous. This is about increasing the trust of the other party that you will be able to take criticism well.

You will be more likely to tell you about a significant issue of personality if you have demonstrated them that you can handle criticism of household chores well.

Easy to take the blame.

Elite being defensive at all costs. Just anticipate that at the moment somebody points out a flaw, you won't feel beautiful. And this is fine. Feeling so is reasonable. Try your best to simply recognize your feedback, thank them for giving it, and explain that you are planning to work on it.

7. Do some micro-traveling

New places and new experiences get us out of our habits and cause us to be more self-conscious.

While I lived in Italy, I recall being shocked initially at how much time people were "wasting" on big, lavish meals — dinner for 3 hours, you are joking!

But after studying Italian culture and being forced into the experience of these long, relaxed meals, it is started to appreciate that alternative attitude towards meals which was more than just a refueling process. And while they don't eat 3-hour dinners regularly, as a result of traveling and time spent in a new environment, perspective on things and their function has changed.

Of course, although regular jet-setting to exotic countries is probably not a viable strategy for most of us, without having to go very far, we can get the self-awareness benefits of travel.

Micro-travel is the simple idea so we can travel on a local scale but still.

 Of starters, whether you live in a big city or urban area, you're probably familiar with your own neighborhood, downtown, and perhaps a couple of other places. But there are still whole neighborhoods in which you haven't invested much, if any, in. That is a micro-travel potential.

Similarly, while two weeks may not be feasible for you in Thailand at the moment, two days at a local state park that you may never have been to.

If we can broaden idea of what traveling means to include still unfamiliar local or nearby locations, we can get many of the benefits of travel — including a boost to our self-awareness — at a fraction of the time or money cost.

8. Learn a new skill

Just as traveling forces us to become more self-aware by throwing ourselves into new situations, learning something new increases awareness of ourselves by forcing us to think and act in new ways.

As adults, we all are set in these ways, and while this leads to some sort of comfort, it also fosters a narrow-mindedness and thinking: when the only things we're doing are things we're good at, it's easy to be lulled into a false sense of security regarding how things work.

The antidote is what is sometimes called The Mind of Beginner. The idea behind beginner's mind is that the brain has to be flexible and see things fresh— like a child — to learn new things. In other words, if we want to cultivate flexibility and freshness within ourselves and the way we see things (i.e. self-awareness), then we should go out of our way to be a beginner.

Either playing the piano, speaking Mandarin, or aqua-coloring, investing in learning a new skill is an essential practice in mental flexibility and self-awareness.

9. Identify cognitive distortions

Cognitive illusions are imprecise perceptions and opinions that affect the way we view things, including ourselves. Just as we can all get into unhelpful physical behaviors (e.g.: nail-biting, late-night snacking, etc.), we all have certain mental habits that don't do us any favors.

For example: Whenever something upsetting happens while I drive — getting cut off, someone taking a parking spot that I wanted— it's a default script running through my mind, What a jerk!

For whatever reason, I have developed a mental habit of calling other drivers by name whenever I get upset on the road. This is a problem because, although other drivers make errors, I do sometimes too.

When I remind myself that the person cutting me off is a dick any time I get cut off and should be a more considerate driver, I may miss the fact that I'm going so far in the passing lane always because I'm talking to my wife and not really mindful of how I'm moving.

The argument is, poor thinking behaviors and self-talk constitute a significant source of a lack of self-awareness. If we can begin to recognize these habits of wrong thinking, we can become more self-conscious — and probably end up feeling better as well.

10.Take the time to explain your principles

 Here's a troubling question: How often do you give time to consider your highest values and ambitions consciously and carefully?

If you're like most of us, the business of everyday life tends to sweep you up in a constant stream of activity without much time for reflection, especially about the most important things.

So, is it shocking then that we have a hard time reaching our targets and achieving happiness when we don't spend any time considering what that might really feel like for us?

It's probably not surprising, however, that we end up following unrealistic targets that culture and society tell us are vital (nice car, big house, slim waistline, Ivy League schools for our babies, etc.) but that we don't actually consider meaningful and satisfying.

A specific form of self-awareness means being aware of the things that really matter to us: Why are we here? What are we waiting for? What makes us truly proud to be able to live a fulfilling life? These are huge questions. And while they seem overwhelming, it's merely because we just don't actually spend a lot of quality time discussing them.

Try this: pull calendar, find a 30-minute time slot once a month (the last Friday of each month I like at 4:30 pm). For this time set up a recurring monthly calendar appointment and call it Clarification of Values. Take out a sheet of paper at this time each month and simply brainstorm ideas and thoughts related to this value question and what you really want. There is no way to do that, right or wrong. What is important is that you give yourself the chance to think about that. You are going to be amazed at what's coming up!

6.3 Spiritual Awakening

Be confident as you view yourself, your environment, and your universe in a different and meaningful way that something inside you can carry out transformation, an ocean of possibility flowing into your existence many are spiritually awakening. By spiritual awakening what do I mean?

Spiritual awakening is a cycle of becoming conscious of our connection to the Almighty. The inner worries have no place on this path, though as we continue to abandon their effects on the lives they will be coming along.

It's a lifelong process to be aware of that relationship. Our awakening journey is not a race, or a competition. It has absolutely nothing to do with the physical world. Though we live in space and time, our awakening is beyond all of this. We're going to come across ourselves as more than just our identities, our families, our bodies. Our awakening takes us into another reality— a reality we can define and understand in time.

To awaken often implies to let go of what you thought to be concrete reality. It is the dissolution of conditioned existence like your beliefs, opinions, and thoughts. You will find that once you come out of the shell of ingrained behavior you don't have your own convictions. Much of your life is lived by other people's beliefs and opinions, and besides that, you cannot state authoritatively who you are. Your awakening challenges your entire identity and allows you to sift through what is really yours and what is not. You must distinguish between real consciousness and programmed consciousness. You will be unfamiliar to the many surprises you encounter through the initial stages, but worry not, comprehension is not far behind. I can't tell you in words that your soul experiences an overwhelming need and a constant ache in its obligation to communicate with you.

The self, the programmed component of you created only by the conditions of this existence, can block the ability of your conscience to pull you into its world of magic and wonders. Your ego is very cunning. It will try to pull you off your path and separate you from your soul, as it doesn't understand the Divine concept. The ego operates on resource limits. It has no clue whatsoever about the misfortunes that visit, the diseases that arise, the heart breaks that cannot heal, the motives behind crime and chaos. By not having access to universal intelligence many of us leave our lives angry, bitter, miserable and dissatisfied.

We have no reference point on why we have endured an injustice, why we have been robbed, why we have been harmed.

When your mind grows, the psyche must experience its inevitable spiritualization. What do I mean by its natural spiritualization?

 The ego will start to understand the essence of the spirit here on earth, and the meaning of the soul. It will slowly begin to change and submit to the will of the mind. Even though the ego gets a base coat, it doesn't need to be demolished but just to improve it. This plays a critical role and needs to be respected.

Be assured that when you perceive yourself, your life, your world in a new and meaningful way, something inside you will bring illumination, an ocean of possibilities pouring into your life, you will become authentic, and thus begin to live the creative life. It is as if for you a mysterious hand of divine origin begins to paint a portrait of your potential and what you are destined to become. The image is a discovery of your personality, intent and reality. If ego and spirit harmoniously combine— this is when the actual life starts.

7: CONCLUSION

The effect of Coaching and improvements* push you to ' end'— the emotions, perceptions, relaxation, joy and fulfillment, strength, knowledge, preference, and possibilities you wanted to accomplish and meet. Achievement is a result, as is happiness, satisfaction, financial safety, holidays, or lifetime or a fulfilling, busy, and fun retirement!

Anyway, what is the goal?! Well, this is the thing you want in the end–the result of your once dreamed-out feeling, behavior, environment, business, career or job, relationship, or lifestyle, even if you never thought you might! Or you wouldn't have taken the step of getting coach help to get you there!

It changes because having new perspectives-how to see things differently, how to think to have no further options or how to feel more happy and healthier in a while!

Anxiety, irritation, pain, or anxiety–the ambiguity that doesn't imply that every day you feel comfortable and happy! You can feel drained and weary from emotionally painful thoughts and feelings, so you need to make changes! Maybe to shake your life, making way for better things to come and be who you know you can be!

If it seems familiar and how you feel, the result you want may be to feel lighter, happier, calmer, and driving your life and career forward! Steadily moving towards a dream, a sensation that is no longer overlooked in your heart and emotions!

The benefits in coaching which are concluded:

A common goal to aim for and move for.

Feel better–calm, going in the right direction.

Feeling happy, stronger, and more comfortable, delighted, you're never feeling anything before or lately!

Get facts and knowledge to make informed choices and successful decisions that help you.

The improvements inside yourself-thoughts in your mind, impulses or desires, to remove pain and restlessness externally and to fulfill your' soul' or spirit' needs, fulfillment and fullness!

Life coaching ultimately make the usual extraordinary.

Through the years, people go through a life or business crisis and have kept their hearts and minds open to positive opportunities. We do not criticize and treat like a survivor. Instead, they keep going, focused on their objectives, and take actions that served each other. They lived their core beliefs and, if necessary, changed their perceptions to remain in the creative flow of life. As a consequence, their lives represent who they are and what they want.

People see dramatic results in themselves and their lives in three to six months of life coaching. However, for those who are challenged to continue growing personally and professionally, long-term coaching services are of value. A person can maintain monthly coaching for several years, return to coaching in high-stress periods, or enter a coaching program. The method of "long-distance" to coaching contributes to a way of life full of honesty, pride, happiness, and peace.

Whether you are interested in short or long-term coaching, here are a few tips to make the most of your life coaching experience: The coach is going to support you.

Engage in a dream, the priorities, and the coaching process. Your coach will allow you to stay focused and deliberate.

Consult with the appropriate instructor behavioral reframes. A change in perception will enable you to take building steps.

Learn to refine new skills.

Focus on a positive outcome, regardless of how turbulent your life is. The mentor will help you in your personal growth to use pressure.

Accept yourself even if your expectations are not met. The mentor tells you of your splendor.

Receive praise and positive feedback from your coach. You will be motivated and trustworthy.

I appreciate your progress one small step at a time. You and your success will be verified by your mentor.

 We can also work with you. You will find in your life pieces of training that you feel more confident, and your life is changing for the better before you know what's happening. People produce remarkable success and draw amazing people and situations into their life while they continue on the road of coaching. It feels magical, but it is the result of efforts done for the job of making positive changes for themselves and their lives and of living with a deep sense of passion and purpose.

8: REFRENCES

1. 10 Ways to Increase Self-Awareness Immediately [With Examples]. Retrieved from **https://nickwignall.com/self-awareness/**

2. 5 Powerful Tips to Overcome Any Challenge. Retrieved from **https://www.guidedmind.com/blog/5-powerful-tips-to-overcome-any-challenge**

3. How to Listen and Build Deeper Connections with People. Retrieved from **https://theartofcharm.com/networking/how-to-listen-and-build-deeper-connections-with-people/**

4. How to Bend Reality - Carla Natalia. Retrieved from **https://carlanatali.com/reality-bender/**

5. Rewrite Your Reality. Retrieved from **https://experiencelife.com/article/rewrite-your-reality/**

6. Huff Post is now a part of Verizon Media. Retrieved from **https://www.huffpost.com/entry/how-to-stop-doubting-your_b_10732946**

7. Create Your Vision: Capturing an Inspiring Picture of the Future. Retrieved from **https://www.eisenhower.me/vision/**

8. Learning to Let Go of Past Hurts: 5 Ways to Move On. Retrieved from **https://psychcentral.com/blog/learning-to-let-go-of-past-hurts-5-ways-to-move-on/**